Picture on Cover

Dr. Denis Burkitt was a medical officer in the British Army during World War II when Britain fought Hitler and the Nazis in Africa. After the war he had a spiritual calling to remain in Africa and become what is known as a "bush doctor" because he particularly sympathized with the indigenous children who needed medical care. He began observing children with large tumors mainly in the face but sometimes on the trunk and extremities. He sought answers as to the cause of the tumors and teamed up with Drs. Anthony Epstein and Yvonne Barr in London who determined that a virus, now called Epstein-Barr virus, caused the tumors. The tumors were labeled "Burkitt's Lymphoma", and this amazing discovery was the first time an infectious agent was found to cause cancer.

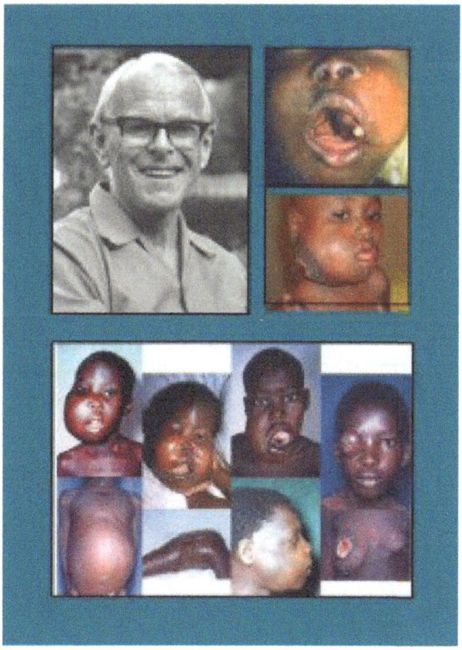

The Epstein-Barr Virus:

A New Factor in the Care of Chronic Pain

By

Forest Tennant, DrPH, MPH, MD

Published by the
Tennant Foundation
West Covina, California

SPONSORS OF THIS BOOK
Tennant Foundation
336-338 S. Glendora Ave.
West Covina, CA 91790-3043
Ph: 626-716-2689
Fax: 626-919-7497
Email: tennantfoundation92@gmail.com

ISBN: 9781955934428
Library of Congress Control Number: 2024919179

U.S. trade bookstores and wholesalers: Please contact
Nancy Kriskovich
Tel: (406)249-2002; or
email snkriskovich@gmail.com

All proceeds from the sale of this book will go to the Medical Study and Education Projects sponsored by the

Tennant Foundation
336-338 S. Glendora Ave.
West Covina, CA 91790-3043
Ph: 626-716-2689
Fax: 626-919-7497
Email: tennantfoundation92@gmail.com

Acknowledgement

Medical Director
Martin J. Porcelli, DO, MPHE, PhD

His anti-viral clinical care has permitted real life observations in chronic pain patients.

Acknowledgement

Ingrid Hollis

Her knowledge of infectious and chronic pain was essential in researching the material for this book.

Publication Development

Rebecca Cholcher-Marino
Nancy Kriskovich

Dedications

Dr. Robert J. Hoagland (Colonel, US Army MC): He was the world's expert on infectious mononucleosis. He was not only an exemplary physician, but a dedicated soldier and medical officer. As I was just entering the US Army as a medical officer, he taught me about infectious mononucleosis and encouraged me to study the disease, provide first class care to our soldiers, and write reports on the disease. This book would never have been written had the colonel not tutored and encouraged me.

Kimrie Donovan, MD: Her insights in living with neurologic disease due to viral infections and her discoveries have been a motivator and "encyclopedia" of knowledge which has helped me write this book.

Authors Notes

I have written this book to highly encourage all concerned parties who deal with chronic and intractable pain to incorporate Epstein-Barr Virus (EBV) testing and treatment into their care plans. Accumulated information makes it clear that EBV reactivation and autoimmunity (EBV R&A) is a causative factor or catalyst in many, if not the majority, of cases of severe chronic and intractable pain. Prevention and treatment measures for EBV R&A are easily done and are a benefit to pain patients.

Reactivation of EBV occurs when the virus changes from its natural, dormant parasitic and harmless state to a disease-producing state. The change occurs when some infection, trauma, fatigue, nutrition, or psychologic stress lowers one's natural immunologic state and allows the "opportunistic" virus to reactivate and develop an autoimmune process that may cause cancer and painful conditions.

When EBV reactivates, it may infiltrate tissues, produce toxins, and develop autoantibodies that cause inflammation, tissue destruction, and pain. Reactivated EBV seems to have a special predilection to inflame and destroy soft tissues like small nerve fibers, membranes, fascia, and intervertebral discs. It also attacks the glial cells of the brain and spinal cord. They become inflamed and destroy nerve tissue around these cells that normally control or "shut off" pain. Hence, constant intractable pain may result.

I wish to recognize the many world class scientists and physicians whose work has made this book possible. All I have done is take one additional step on the foundation they built. No one makes a scientific or medical discovery and advancement without building on the work of others. The story and journey behind my efforts salute the names of Fothergill, Coburn, Burkitt, Hoagland, Epstein, Sumaya, Barr, Henle, Watkins, Apkarian, and Teitelbaum. I send my deep gratitude and many thanks.

It is my hope that the care of severe, chronic and intractable pain patients will now include EBV testing and treatment as I have personally observed great reduction in pain and suffering when EBV R&A is curtailed.

Prologue

The Epstein-Barr virus (EBV) is a parasitic virus that is carried by over 95% of adults. After its initial activation and entrance into the human body during childhood or early adult years, it normally remains dormant and harmless in lymphocytes and nasopharyngeal membranes. EBV can reactivate from its latent state during times of stress which can be infectious, traumatic, nutritional, fatigue, or psychological. Once reactivated, EBV may produce an autoimmune process and/or infiltrate tissues to cause some cancers and a variety of chronic and intractable pain conditions.

Every person who has a severe, chronic or intractable pain condition is highly advised to determine if EBV R&A are a causative factor in their painful condition. Failure to control and contain EBV R&A may allow the painful condition to deteriorate and result in incapacitation, early death, or other tragic consequence. Testing and treatment measures have recently been identified, and, in the experience of the author, have helped reduce pain and suffering.

Contents

1. Introduction

On April 18, 2018, the results of a far-reaching scientific study on the Epstein-Barr Virus (EBV) were announced.[37,38] The study garnered little media attention. Most likely because EBV has been around a long time, and, in the minds of both medical practitioners and lay public, EBV is the "old kissing disease" that is rather harmless. To me, however, this study was most needed and welcome. There had not been a single major advance in the science and understanding of intractable pain (IP) for over a decade. At that time, some brilliant researchers found that IP often occurred after the glial cells in the brain and spinal cord activated, produced neuroinflammation, and decimated tissues that normally prevent the development of IP.[111,112] The question remained, however, as to what caused the glial cells to activate in the first place?

Specifically, Dr. John Harley and his researchers at the Veteran's and Children's Hospitals in Cincinnati, Ohio found that an EBV protein known as EBNA-2 (Epstein-Barr nuclear antigen) interacted with genes that are associated with the development of multiple sclerosis, rheumatoid arthritis, systemic lupus, inflammatory bowel disease, type 1 diabetes, juvenile arthritis, and celiac disease.[37,38] All of these conditions are known to cause significant disability, functional impairments, and, in some cases, IP. Support for the Harley study was done soon after by Bjornevik and colleagues who, in 2022, published a seminal report in Science.[12] They found that 955 active-duty military young adults who developed multiple sclerosis had negative EBV serum antibodies before their disease but converted to EBV positive after the onset of their disease.

Shortly after these two studies, some additional ones forced me to immediately begin to intently study EBV in IP patients. These studies showed that EBV will activate glial cells in the central nervous system (CNS-brain and spinal cord) and create neuroinflammation.[50,51,52,64] The obvious question was whether EBV had been causing glial cell activation, immense suffering, and premature deaths in IP all along. These new scientific discoveries were the incentive I needed. I had been collecting and analyzing viral test results in chronic pain patients for years, but I had come to a roadblock. Although EBV showed up in all my testing, I wasn't sure which virus was most likely the one that caused glial cell activation and neuroinflammation, which is a key step in the development of intractable pain.[49,69,106] I now had my marching orders.

Over the last three years my daily investigations into EBV and pain care have convinced me that many, if not most, persons with both IP and severe chronic pain (SCP) are at least partially the result of EBV R&A. Some other viruses may be involved with IP, but EBV is usually the leader. Intractable pain (IP) is defined as constant incurable pain that may produce cardiovascular, respiratory, endocrine, and metabolic complications.[99,100] It is usually preceded by chronic pain (CP) which is defined as a pain that persists longer than the usual healing time of ninety days and which requires daily medication for relief.[32]

As this book is being written, countless persons have IP or SCP and don't really know how they developed their maladies or why they worsen and do not improve even with the best of modern medical care. Millions of people have literally awakened one day with a severe back, muscle, or head pain and wondered what they "caught." EBV may be the cause of their lifetime of grief and misery. Anyone who believes EBV couldn't possibly be the relatively harmless "kissing disease", and the cause of their SCP should carefully look at the children's pictures on the front cover of this book. If EBV can cause cancer and eat away one's jaw, leg, or breast it can certainly eat away the discs in your spine, nerves in your groin, or glial cells in your brain.[20-24] The good news is that testing to determine EBV reactivation and autoimmunity (EBV R&A) has been developed and medical measures have been identified to contain and control the virus. Information to date has clearly shown this author that pain patients enhance their care with some specific prevention and medical measures that contain and control EBV R&A.

This book is intended to present the history, scientific developments, and some suggestions on testing and treatment of EBV R&A. It is jointly written for both patients and medical practitioners. Regardless of whether you are a patient with SCP or IP or a medical practitioner who wants to help, this book will at least give you some background, rationale, and preliminary control measures to improve pain care.

2. Epstein-Barr Activation, Reactivation and Autoimmunity Defined

It is critical that persons with IP or SCP and their medical practitioners understand the terms, activation, reactivation and autoimmunity in order to control and contain EBV.

The first EBV activation almost always occurs before adulthood.[25,26,108] EBV usually invades the body in the first two years of life or during an episode of infectious mononucleosis as a teenager or young adult. In infancy, EBV activation usually resembles a common cold or "sniffles." After its initial activation and entry into the human body, it becomes a carrier and parasite in throat membranes and lymphocytes (B class which makes antibodies rather than the T class which is the "helper" class). The parasitic state is usually harmless and known as a carrier, dormant, or latent state.

Reactivation is defined as "a change from a dormant, carrier, or latent state to one in which the virus begins to duplicate and becomes an active infectious agent that can produce diseases including cancer and painful conditions." EBV will reactivate especially under stressful conditions.[60,61,64,65,92] Viral reactivation is hardly a new concept as everyone has witnessed it. The herpes class of viruses are well known parasites in the human body.[72,93,109] They commonly reactivate at some point after their initial activation and entry into the body to produce a disease condition.[77,85] Herpes simplex number one reactivates to cause blisters in and around the mouth and lips. Herpes simplex number two reactivates and forms blisters on the genitalia. Herpes zoster may reactivate to cause a skin rash known as "shingles."[15] EBV is a member of the herpes class and has been given the number four. All the herpes viruses including cytomegalovirus may accompany EBV in causing disease and pain.[1]

Once reactivated, EBV can cause tissue inflammation, destruction, and pain by infiltrating tissues, producing toxic or poisonous substances, or initiate a process known as autoimmunity.[27,108] Autoimmune disease is defined as "a disease in which the person's own tissues are mistaken by an autoantibody to act like an outside harmful invader such as a bacteria or virus.[11] Simply defined autoimmunity is "a disease process that attacks and destroys tissue by an autoantibody."[33-35] There are about 100 different diseases which are classified as autoimmune. Most are quite rare. The best-known autoimmune diseases are rheumatoid arthritis, systemic lupus erythematosus, Sjogren's syndrome, Hashimoto's thyroiditis, psoriasis, and ankylosing spondylitis. The attached tables list the autoimmune diseases and cancers that have been associated with EBV reactivation.

In the early years of the last century neither EBV nor infectious mononucleosis were considered to have any connection to autoimmunity. By 1974 it was clear that EBV and infectious mononucleosis (IM) produced autoantibodies.[94] Later studies showed that reactivated EBV also produce autoantibodies.[82] The lymphocytes which harbor the virus may become a plasma cell if EBV reactivates. Autoantibodies are produced by the plasma cells and are carried in the antibody known as Epstein-Barr nuclear antigen antibody (abbreviated EBNA). The virus may also infiltrate normal tissues and possibly form an autoantibody against the tissue. Simply put, researchers have identified multiple ways that EBV reactivation may induce EBV autoimmunity. Consequently, reactivation of EBV can rightfully be called an autoimmune disease.

EBV autoimmunity can be clinically presumed to be present if there is a significant elevation of its two protective antibodies (EBNA) and virus capsid antibody (VCA) as well as the presence of two or more painful conditions which are found in the later chapter "Multi-Site, Migratory Pain Disease." In summary, it is recommended that there be both laboratory and clinical evidence before the term EBV R&A is applied to a patient.

The term "causative factor" is used here to indicate that EBV may be one of multiple factors that cause painful conditions. The tables in this chapter summarize the known cancer and autoimmune diseases linked to EBV.

A major problem with autoimmunity is that it may not be totally eliminated despite aggressive medical treatment. This is clearly the experience, for example, with rheumatoid arthritis and systemic lupus.[47] Once its presence is determined, ongoing measures to suppress it are well-advised, but cure may not be possible.

In summary, EBV R&A may be a causative factor in a variety of cancers and painful conditions.

TABLE

AUTOIMMUNE DISORDERS THAT HAVE EBV REACTIVATION AND AUTOIMMUNITY AS A CAUSATIVE FACTOR

Rheumatoid arthritis
Grave's disease (hyperthyroidism)
Hashimoto's thyroiditis
Systemic lupus erythematosus
Multiple sclerosis
Inflammatory bowel syndrome
Celiac disease
Non-infectious hepatitis
Type 1 diabetes
Polyneuropathy
Sjogren's syndrome

TABLE

CANCERS IN WHICH EBV IS A CAUSATIVE FACTOR

Lymphomas
Nasopharyngeal
Gastric
Hodgkin's

3. The Beginning

It may sound strange, but the beginning starts in the 1930's when Adolf Hitler and his Nazi's embarked on a plan to rule the world and exterminate all Jews. For starters a young Jewish man named Werner Henle graduated in medicine from the University of Heidelberg, Germany, in 1934. He had a Jewish grandfather named Jacob Henle who was a famous 19th century anatomist. Consequently, young Dr. Henle had his career blocked and perhaps life threatened. He immigrated to the US in 1936 and arguably became the world's top virologist. In 1968 he and his virologist wife discovered that EBV caused infectious mononucleosis (IM).[41]

In 1941 Hitler and the Italians invaded Africa. In this same year a young British surgeon, Denis Burkitt, was commissioned into the Royal Army Medical Corp. Dr. Burkitt went on to arguably benefit society as much or more than any physician in the past century. In 2005 Dr. Erle Robertson, who worked with Dr. Werner Henle wrote a seminal book on EBV. It contains most of Dr. Burkitt's biography. In 1970, Dr. Burkitt, himself, wrote a book on his discoveries, and much is repeated here.

Dr. Burkitt was born in 1911 in Enniskillen, a picturesque town in Northern Ireland. Sadly, at the age of 11, young Denis suffered an injury that left him blind in one eye. Denis later decided to become an engineer and enrolled at Trinity College in Dublin, Ireland. He joined the University Christian Society which gave new meaning to his life, and he resolved to become a missionary. Fortunately for the discoveries he would make in his later life, he shared a room with a medical student. His roommate talked about medicine and influenced Denis to become a doctor rather than an engineer.

After joining the Royal Army Medical Corps at age 30, he served for about two years in Southern England with the 219 Field Ambulance Unit. In 1943 he was sent to East Africa with the British Colonial African Troops. Here he was stationed in Kenya and Somaliland where British troops campaigned against the Italians. While on occasional leave, Dr. Burkitt visited Uganda. At that time Uganda was often described as "the pearl of Africa" because it was a prosperous and peaceful country. It had Christian beliefs and activity which appealed to Dr. Burkitt's deeply religious convictions. He decided, at the time, that after the war he would devote his life to helping the people of Uganda, particularly, the children who desperately needed medical care.

After demobilization and the end of the war in 1946, he applied to the British Colonial Office to join its Medical Service in Uganda. He was accepted and began duty as a government servant and not as a volunteer missionary as is sometimes erroneously stated. Dr. Burkitt's first assignment was in Lira, Lanza District where he was in sole medical charge of a population of about 300,000 with nothing more than a 100-bed bush hospital to cover all medical and surgical needs. Dr. Burkitt wasn't just a doctor with a missionary zeal. He was a great observer and data collector. His first contribution to published medical science was a data collection of 200 cases of hydrocele which is a fluid collection that surrounds the testes in the scrotum.[18] Almost all of the cases came from East rather than West Lanzo district, so he correctly determined that the cases were caused by bilharziasis which is a long, threadlike worm that can enter the body through mosquito bites and block blood vessels and lymphatic drainage.

In 1957 Dr. Burkitt was working in Mulago Hospital in Kampala, the Capital of Uganda. He was consulted by a colleague about a child with a puzzling swelling of the jaw. Dr. Burkitt didn't think it was an infection or a cancer, and he kept meticulous notes on his care along with photographs. Shortly afterwards, quite by chance, while visiting another hospital, he noticed another child with swelling of the jaw. The boy also had tumors in his abdomen. Dr. Burkitt realized that these two cases had to be the same disease but caused by something quite extraordinary. He had an inquiring mind, and when he returned to his home hospital in Kampala, he researched their records for children with jaw tumors. Low and behold he found records of several similar cases. Both of the cases he had personally seen plus the hospital records revealed that the children, both boys and girls, had jaw tumors and also may have had tumors in other parts of their body. He concluded that he had discovered a heretofore, unrealized childhood tumor complex that had a single cause that was common in Ugandan children in their first decade of life.

In 1958 Dr. Burkitt published his findings in the British Journal of Surgery. He called the tumors "sarcoma" which is now regarded as cancer.[19] His article and findings created almost zero interest. After all, who could possibly be interested in jaw tumors of Ugandan children? Not to be deterred, Dr. Burkitt teamed up with a pathologist, G.T. O'Connor, who looked at tumor cells under a microscope and determined that they were a lymphoma. This meant that the children's lymph nodes had experienced something that caused their cells to go "wild," duplicate, and form a destructive tissue mass. Drs. Burkitt and O'Connor published their findings in 1961 in the journal, Cancer.[20] The report had this title: "Malignant Lymphoma in African Children: A Clinical Syndrome." Although this report didn't implicate a virus, it caught the attention of some cancer scientists and researchers. Since the tumors were in a localized geographic area, a general belief by many, including Dr. Burkitt, hypothesized that a vector or insect must spread the disease. Regardless, Dr. Burkitt, to his great credit, had not only recognized the disease but attempted to determine its origin and cause. Following his publication with Dr. O'Connor in 1961, enough parties recognized that these childhood tumors were a major medical discovery and invited Dr. Burkitt to speak about his findings. Enter Dr. Epstein.

The Epstein-Barr Virus:

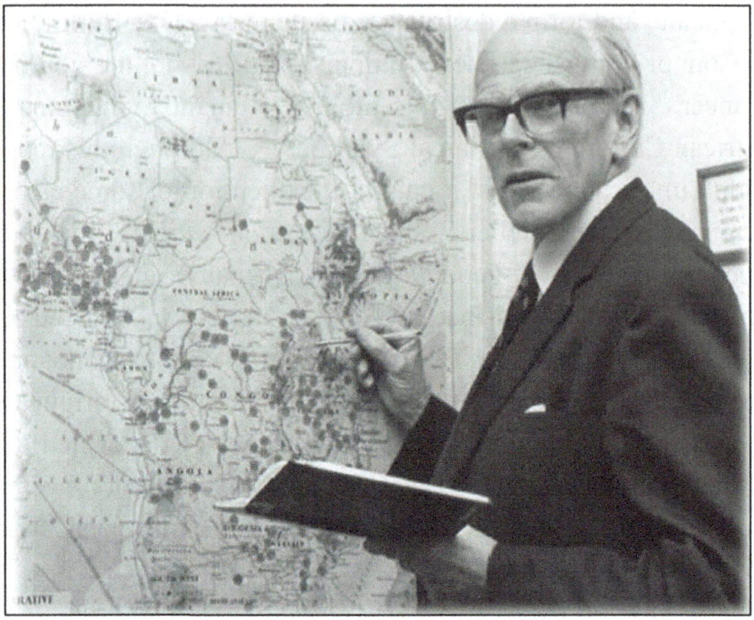

Dr. Denis Burkitt, who discovered the lymphoma from which Drs. Epstein and Barr isolated the virus, is shown giving a lecture. He is pointing to areas in Africa where he found children with EBV tumors.

The following photographs are examples of Burkitt's lymphoma in children and teenagers between the ages of five and twenty. The cause is the Epstein-Barr Virus. Tumors were predominantly on the face, but some were on other parts of the body.

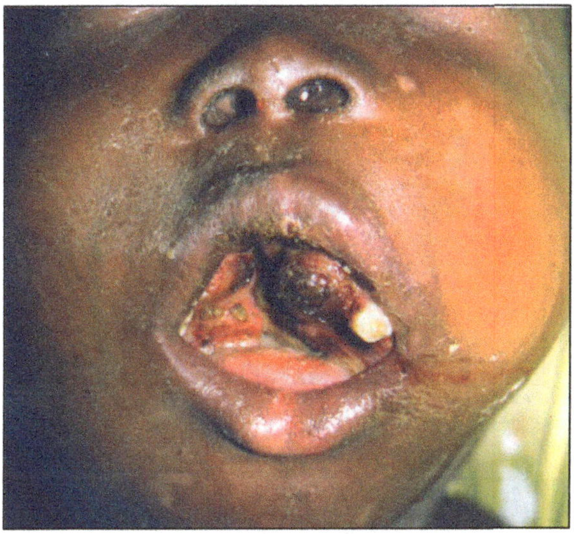

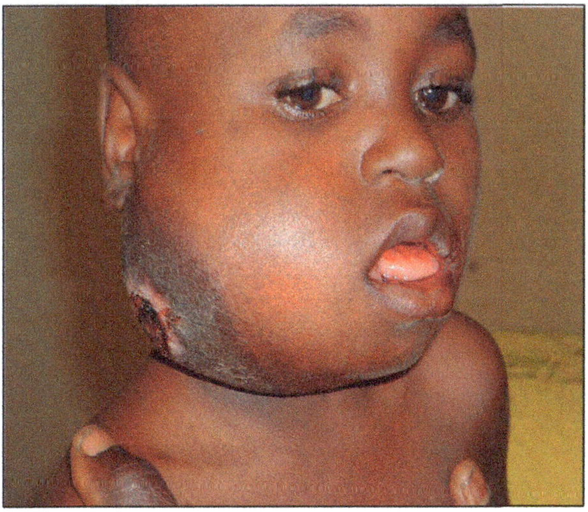

The Epstein-Barr Virus:

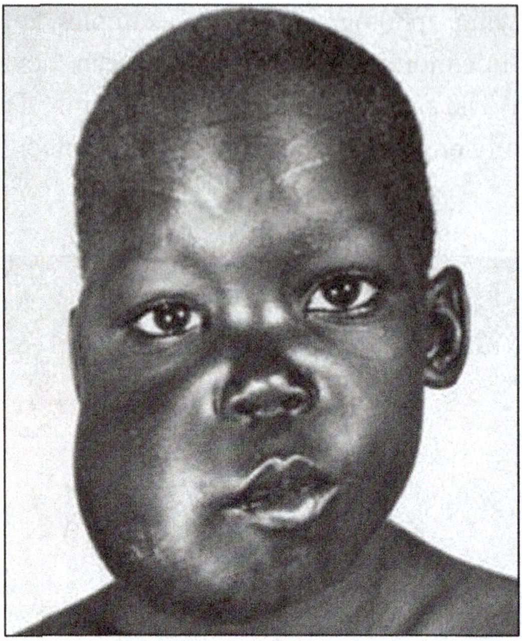

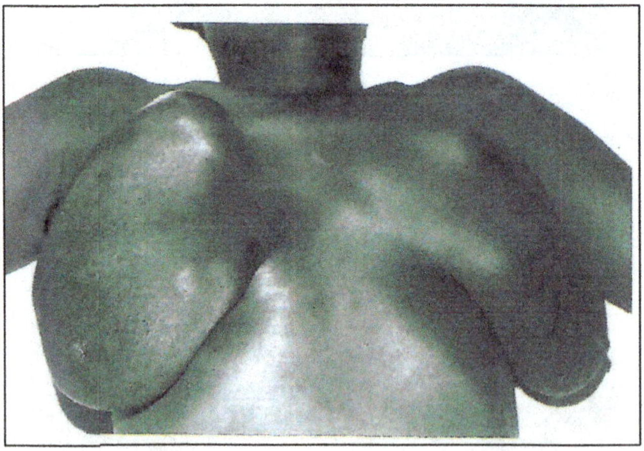

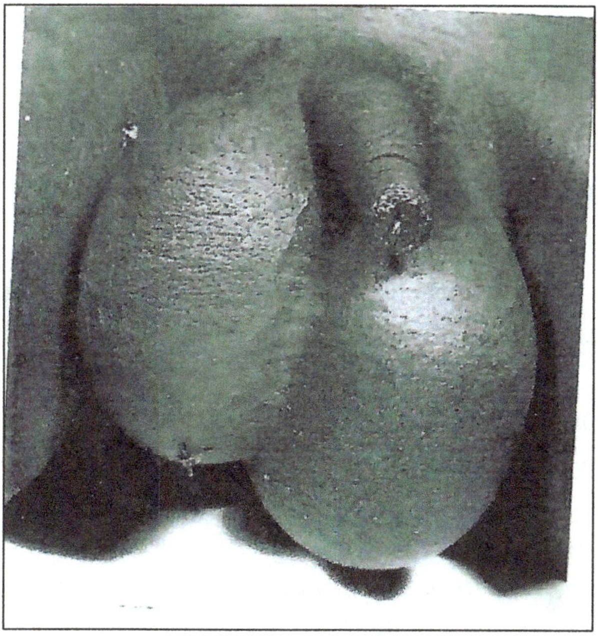

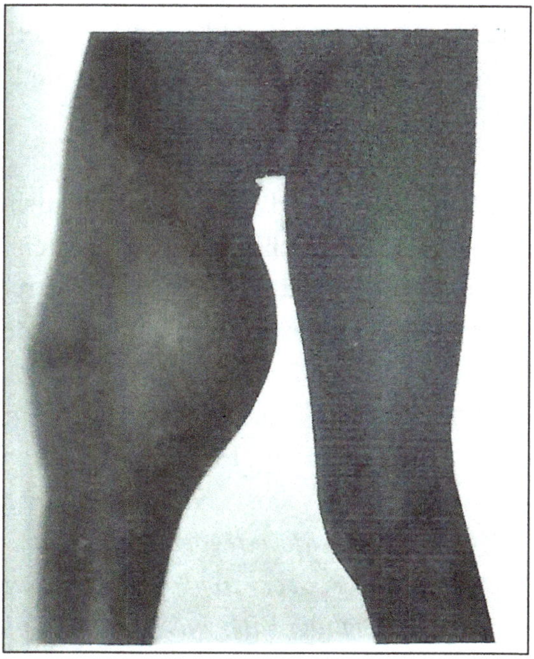

4. The Epstein-Barr Discovery: A Virus Causes Cancer

Dr. M. Anthony Epstein was the right man, at the right time, and in the right place to discover that EBV caused Dr. Burkitt's tumors. The acclaim given to Dr. Epstein is historically well placed as his discovery was the first to document that an infectious agent could cause a cancer.[31]

For the record, Dr. Epsteinwas born in London on May 18, 1921. He lived to be 102 years old, passing earlier this year, 2024. He became a pathologist and a professor. He ascended the professional ranks to become head of the pathology department at the University of Bristol. Besides being a great scientist, Dr. Epstein was personable and an excellent leader. As with all great scientists, he had a curious mind and was a good writer who could convey his discoveries.

He received many awards and was made a British Knight in 1991 earning the title "Sir Michael Anthony Epstein." As with most famous people and great discoveries, many renditions of his discovery that EBV causes cancer contain inaccuracies and even fraudulent material. In 2005 Dr. Epstein personally wrote a detailed chronology of his discovery in the seminal book, Epstein Barr Virus, edited by Erle S. Robertson. In Dr. Epstein's words he wrote his story, *"because of the persistence of inaccuracies it was considered worthwhile in the thirty-fifth anniversary year of the discovery to provide a definitive history of the circumstances in which EBV was first recognized."*

What follows here is close to verbatim his history of the discovery. Dr. E.S. Robertson's exquisite book recorded Dr. Epstein's personal rendition of the facts. Before meeting Dr. Burkitt, Dr. Epstein had an interest in and believed that viruses could possibly cause cancer. During the 1950's and in the early part of his career, he studied and published extensively on a virus called "Rous" which appeared to possibly cause a cancer called sarcoma. At this time the world was generally oblivious and uninterested in either Drs. Burkitt or Epstein's work and beliefs. The idea that a virus could cause cancer was a far-fetched, ridiculous idea. Dr. Epstein, in his biography, says only about a dozen scientists world-wide in the 1960's considered virus-induced cancer a topic of interest.

As good luck would have it, Dr. Burkitt had a connection to the Academic Surgical Unit at the Middlesex Hospital where Dr. Epstein headquartered. When Dr. Burkitt returned to England on home leave he would customarily be invited to lecture staff and students on his experiences treating the exotic and bizarre cases he encountered in the developing country of Uganda. As further good luck, Dr. Burkitt was scheduled to give a talk on March 22, 1961, which he titled "The Commonest Children's Cancer in Tropical Africa: A Hitherto Unrecognized Syndrome."

Dr. Epstein relates that he "quite randomly" saw the announcement about the talk and for reasons he didn't quite recall decided to attend the lecture. He attended the lecture and was "electrified" from the start by the strange nature and progression of the disease as well as its geographic location. Dr. Epstein, even before Dr. Burkitt finished his talk, resolved to investigate the tumor for unusual viruses.

The Epstein-Barr Virus:

Anyone seeing the pictures in this book would have to be "electrified" and wonder how such a disease could exist.

Interestingly, Dr. Epstein in his biography made a distinct point of the lack of interest in viruses in the early 1960's. In London Dr. Burkitt gave, in a large lecture theatre at the Royal College of Surgeons, a presentation which was only attended by twelve people. Afterward Dr. Burkitt shrugged off his disappointment when he said he was "just an unknown bush surgeon." Dr. Epstein was not deterred and says he eternally kept Dr. Burkitt's lecture announcement at the front of his EBV file.

After Dr. Burkitt's lecture, he and Dr. Epstein got together and agreed to collaborate. Both Drs. Epstein and Burkitt felt initially that a vector such as a mosquito, which was known to carry and spread malaria and yellow fever, must be involved.

They agreed to have tissue samples taken from the children's tumors and sent from Uganda to London to be analyzed by Dr. Epstein and his assistants. Dr. Epstein made a trip to Uganda to work out the details. To pay for the trip he needed financial assistance that he said was difficult to obtain due to "politics at the very top of the British establishment concerned with cancer research." This author, in studying Dr. Epstein's leadership and career, has determined that he had a most pleasant personality and persuasive way to gain cooperation from the parties he had to encounter in order to accomplish his monumental achievements.

Beginning in late 1961 and 1962 tumor samples were regularly obtained and shipped from Uganda to England. For almost two years Dr. Epstein attempted to both find a virus in the tumor samples and/or grow a virus from the tumors.

His plan and hope to grow a laboratory tumor from a human lymphocyte tumor was a daunting task that had never been accomplished. He and his assistants set out to grow a Burkitt lymphoma in "a test tube." They tried, in vain, to grow a tumor by use of what they called "floating lymphoma fragments, in plasma clots and fragments on rafts." They inoculated tumor extracts into various kinds of cell cultures including embryonic eggs and newborn mice. He also began working with the newly invented electron microscope hoping to spot a virus that grew in a cell culture. After two years of multiple techniques and efforts, Dr. Epstein and his team of assistants could neither grow the tumor nor spot a virus in the tumors. Dr. Epstein admitted that two years of fruitless efforts without results were "depressing and alarming at a particularly insecure stage of my career."

At a low point of despair for Dr. Epstein and his staff, an unexpected event occurred on Friday, December 3, 1963. A flight from Kampala, Uganda carrying tumor samples was directed to Manchester due to fog and didn't reach London until several hours after its scheduled time of arrival. The tissue was, as usual, floating in guinea pig serum and saline transit fluid but the fluid was unusually cloudy. It was initially assumed that the sample was ruined by bacterial contamination during the long-delayed flight.

Before discarding what he originally thought to be a ruined sample, Dr. Epstein decided to look at a drop of the turbid fluid under a regular, light microscope. Much to his astonishment, he saw a large number of round, viable looking, free-floating tumor cells that had been shaken free during the delayed flight. Dr. Epstein immediately recalled a study by a Yale researcher named G.A. Fischer, who had reported that the method to grow a "test tube tumor" was to use single cells rather than tissue fragments.[33] It didn't take Dr. Epstein long to shift courses.

Dr. Epstein was also aware of a reported study by RA Bonor and colleagues who had been able to grow chicken tumors in a test tube or dish by use of single cells from a tumor.[13] He managed to obtain a $45,000 grant from the US National Cancer Institute which allowed him to recruit Yvonne Barr and Bert Achon, as assistants. Dr. Epstein and his new talented assistants used a single cell technique to grow a Burkitt's lymphoma in a test tube. Their perseverance and scientific professionalism to build on other's work paid off. Burkitt's lymphoma had grown in the lab and the virus grew out. Drs. Epstein and Barr published their results in the prestigious journal Lancet in 1964.[31] Ever since their discovery and publication in 1964, the virus has been called Epstein-Barr. The laboratory technique to grow tumors cells and identify an offending virus which was developed by Dr. Epstein and his assistants is still standard today.

Drs. Epstein and Barr made a monumental discovery: an infectious agent can cause cancer. We all owe them deep gratitude. Science moves slow, but we now know the EBV virus they discovered is ubiquitous and can be a major, causative factor in many cancers and painful conditions.

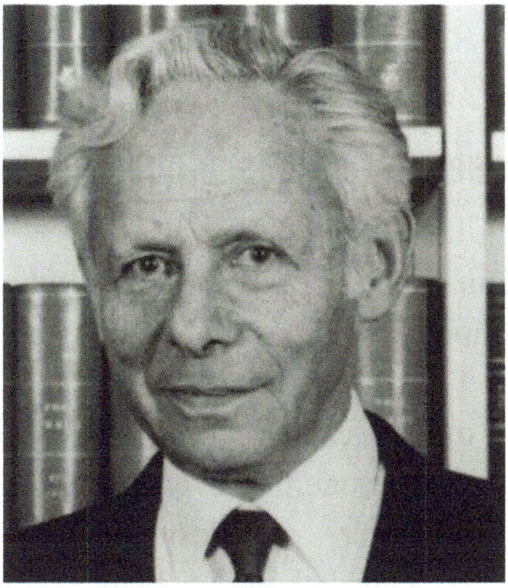

Dr. Anthony Epstein

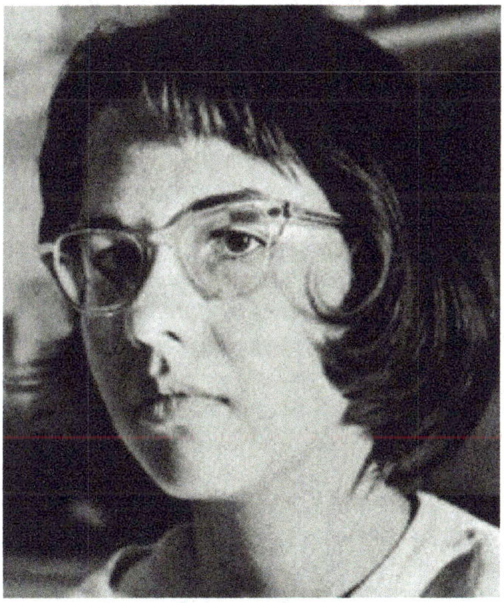

Dr. Yvonne Barr

These scientists discovered that a virus caused Burkitt's lymphoma. The virus is named after them. It is now recognized that EBV can cause cancer and painful disease.

5. EBV Causes Infectious Mononucleosis

After Dr. Epstein found a virus in cell cultures derived from Burkitt's lymphoma, he encountered disbelief from the scientific world. First, it wasn't yet accepted that you could take tissues from a human cancer and regrow the cancer in a laboratory. Second, no one had even heard or believed that a virus could cause cancer. Dr. Epstein clearly knew that he needed a second laboratory to duplicate his methods and results in order that his discoveries be scientifically accepted. Initially he contacted two leading British herpes virologists, but neither was interested. He therefore contacted two old virologist friends, Werner and Gertrude Henle in Philadelphia, PA.

The story and life of Werner and Gertrude Henle are hardly known to anyone except to those persons who follow viral and autoimmune research. Simply stated, to those of us in the research world of viral diseases, the Henle's are "unsung heroes."

As noted in the "Beginning" chapter, Werner Henle graduated from medical school at the University of Heidelberg, Germany in 1934. This timing coincided with the rise of the Nazi era. Werner had a grandfather who was a famous Jewish anatomist in the 19th century. Consequently, as a Jewish physician, the Nazi's blocked him from establishing a medical career in Germany. He, therefore, immigrated to the United States for employment and possibly to save his life. The following year Gertrude Sopinger also graduated from the same medical school. Having known Werner for some time, she came to the

United States in 1937 and became Gertrude Henle the day after arrival. The two went on to become known as the "esteemed virologist couple" and the "world's best" as they not only discovered that EBV caused IM but made many discoveries that either underpin or are practiced in medicine today.[39-43]

The Henle's didn't need a lot of coaxing to accept Dr. Epstein's plea to duplicate his work. In 1963, even before the famed EBV discovery and publication of it by Drs. Epstein and Barr, they had been encouraged to study Burkitt's lymphoma by C Everett Koop, MD. Dr. Koop, at the time, was surgeon-in-general of the Children's Hospital in Philadelphia. Dr. Koop later became one of the most popular and charismatic surgeon generals of the United States. He visited Africa in 1963, returned home, and reportedly told the Henle's "If you really want to work on a tumor which is most likely caused by a virus, you should work on Burkitt's lymphoma."

After the Henle's agreed to collaborate with Dr. Epstein and his team, the events and accomplishments that ensued are truly a tribute to science and the dedication of many people who were involved with the scientific discoveries that were to follow. Shortly after the Henle's started their EBV journey, Dr. Harold Van Hanson applied to work with the Henle's in a postdoctoral position in their lab. He was accepted and flew from Germany to Philadelphia and began work on EBV in their lab on January 2, 1966. Dr. Van Hanson wrote a detailed and most complementary account of the Henle efforts in Dr. Erle Robertson's seminal book, "Epstein-Barr Virus." My writing here is extracted from his detailed account of their efforts. The Henle's, along with Dr. Van Hanson and other members of their team, developed antibody tests for EBV and clearly proved that EBV caused Burkitt's lymphoma. They gave Drs. Epstein and

Barr the hard evidence they needed to prove that a virus could cause cancer.[49,50]

The discovery most accredited to the Henle's is that EBV causes infectious mononucleosis. Dr. Hanson incorporated Dr. Werner Henle's account of how they discovered that EBV was the long sought-after cause of IM. In Wener Henle's words,

> *"The answer to our search for an illness caused by EBV came quite unexpectedly right in our laboratory when one of our technicians reported ill in August 1967. She was seronegative for EBV and had been a frequent, more or less willing, donor for leukocytes for EBV. Our technician returned to work five days later but developed under our eyes a rubella-like look. Her physician had considered either rubella or IM as probable diagnosis. We obtained blood from her for serologic tests as well as yet another leukocyte culture thinking more of rubella than IM. The heterophile antibody test, however, turned out to be positive. The rash was then not due to rubella but ampicillin which she had received and which for unknown reasons can be the cause of a rash in IM patients. We noted next with astonishment that our technician had developed antibodies to EBV since the last time we tested her and observed in due course her leukocytes which formerly never survived in culture grew this time into a permanent lymphoblastoid cell line with a small percentage of EBV-producing cells. These were the first exciting clues that EBV was the long-sought cause of IM. It was fortunate that we never took our summer vacation in August since in our absence this event would probably have passed unnoticed."*

In a subsequent collaborative study with two researchers, Jim Niederman and Bob McCollum, "pre-sera" was taken from college students who later developed IM. Sera obtained after the infection showed the presence of EBV antibodies, so this finding left no doubt that EBV caused IM.[75]

The Henle team conducted and published many studies on EBV. Two of their early studies have great relevance to CP and IP. In 1970 and 1971, the Henle's, along with other collaborators, found extremely high EBV antibody titers in Hodgkin's disease and chronic lymphocytic leukemia.[3,42,56,57] The Henle's interpreted this to be a reactivation of latent EBV infection. The concept of EBV reactivation, from the latent dormant, or carrier state, was a foreign concept at the time. Interestingly, physicians in the late 1800's, believed in "autoinfection" which they thought was a disease that occurred due to an infectious agent that normally lived in the intestine.[36] This early belief that a parasite in the body could migrate and cause disease, however, is basically the mechanism whereby EBV causes cancers and painful diseases.

Within a period of slightly more than 20 years, this dedicated couple collaborated with numerous laboratories around the world and published approximately 300 manuscripts. When Werner Henle died on July 6, 1987, at the age of seventy-six, his wife Gertrude of 50 years retired from her most active and contributory career in virology. Some 30 to 40 years have passed, but their pioneering work has already been a great benefit to millions of people.

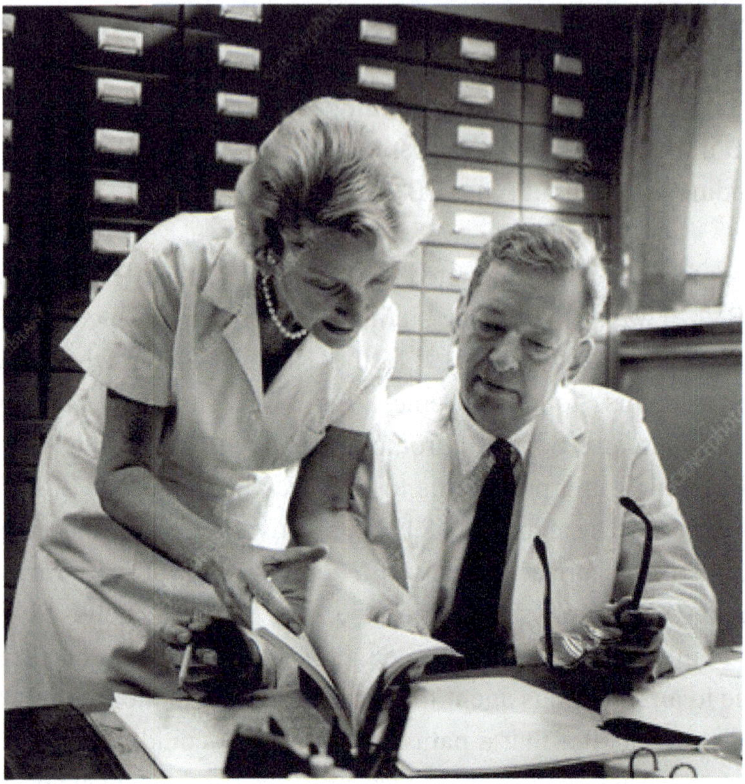

Drs Werner and Gertrude Henle were considered the world's top virologists in the mid-twentieth century. They both graduated from medical school in Germany and came to the United States and married just prior to the start of World War II. They confirmed the work of Drs. Epstein and Barr and went on to develop diagnostic antibody tests that are used today and discovered how the Epstein-Barr virus causes mononucleosis, cancer, and painful conditions.

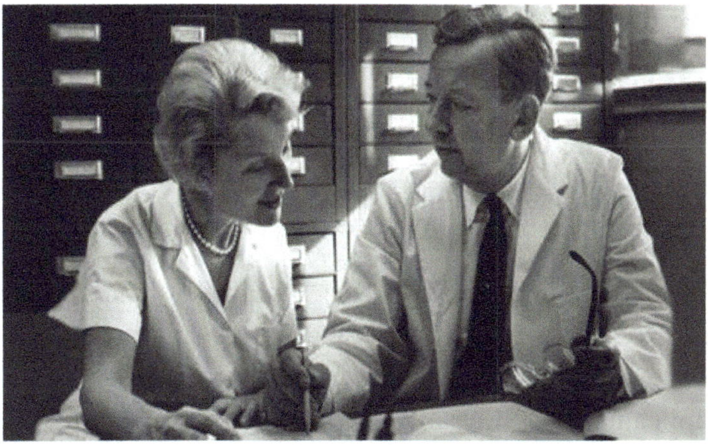

Drs. Werner and Gertrude Henle collaborating in their lab.

6. Search for Cure and Complications of Infectious Mononucleosis

At about the same time that Drs. Burkitt, Epstein, and Henle were investigating EBV and cancer, some physicians in the United States were vigorously studying IM and its complications. IM was still often referred to as glandular fever which was a name applied to it in the 1800's. The disease seemed to be more prevalent after World War II. It was a contagious and widespread disease, especially in college dormitories and military barracks.[35] The cause was unknown and not discovered and reported by Werner and Gertrude Henle until 1968. Complications of IM such as hepatitis and pneumonia sometimes occurred and caused hospitalization and intense medical care. Fatalities were rare.

The unquestionable physician authority on IM during the 1950's and 60's was Colonel Robert J. Hoagland, MD.[45] He was a career Army medical officer and was assigned to the US Military Academy Hospital (West Point) as Chief of the Department of Medicine in 1946. He saw many cadets with the disease and began to study it. He was aware that IM was primarily a disease of college age persons and there had been an outbreak of IM at the US Naval Academy as well as several colleges. Naturally, the Army had a keen interest in IM as soldiers had to be constantly fit for duty. Dr. Hoagland kept immaculate records, and in August 1952 published data on 56 cases.[45] In this report he established firm criteria to diagnose the disease. One had to have the physical findings indicative of a throat infection with swollen cervical (neck) lymph nodes, a positive serologic test known as a heterophile, and a preponderance of lymphocytes in the blood. He also, in the report, described typical eyelid swelling seen in patients with IM. This became known, even today, as the "Hoagland sign."[14]

Amazingly, in 1967, at just about the same time the Henles discovered the cause of IM, he published a seminal book simply titled "Infectious Mononucleosis." This was his detailed account of 500 consecutive cases of IM that he personally treated. Dr. Hoagland's experience took place before 1968 when the Henles reported that EBV caused IM. There isn't a single word about EBV, Burkitt's lymphoma, or reactivation in Dr. Hoagland's book. The book, however, is a classic. Seldom do physicians get the opportunity to learn from a large, documented series of cases. Any physician wishing to study EBV or IM will find this book invaluable.

In June 1966, I graduated with an MD degree from the University of Kansas. The only thing I recall being taught about IM in medical school was that it was the "kissing disease." The professor who gave the lecture said he would rather admit he had syphilis or gonorrhea because IM was only contracted by kissing and usually transmitted by women of nefarious character. It should be pointed out that the origin of the "kissing" label is somewhat obscure, but IM was common among young adults who dated a lot, so this label seemed appropriate. Epidemiologic studies have shown, however, that only about 5 to 10% of IM cases could possibly be traced to kissing.

During medical school I accepted a US Army scholarship with the quid pro quo that I would serve at least three years on active duty after I graduated. Knowing that a long stint in the Army was forthcoming, I guided my medical studies into infectious disease and physical fitness. The Vietnam War was heating up and so was the new ability to Med-E-Vac (helicopter and air transport) injured soldiers to centers for trauma surgery or treatment of infectious disease. The days of mobile army surgical hospitals (MASH) were essentially over. The Army needed docs who knew a lot about infectious diseases and physical fitness. This suited my tastes and education.

In 1965, the medical school system in the United States changed how graduating students could select their one-year internship following graduation. You could pick a specialty for your internship, and I picked internal medicine as the best way to study infectious diseases and cardiac fitness. The new internship selection program had the student sign up for three internships. I signed up for ones in Fort Worth, Saint Paul, and Louisville. Like the football or basketball draft, you had to go where selected. Louisville picked me. Neither I nor my future wife, Miriam, had ever been to Louisville but the idea of seeing the thoroughbred horses and the Kentucky Derby was a lure along with our belief that Louisville General Hospital would be a great place for Army preparation. Miriam loved horses and, in fact, even rode one to school while growing up on an Eastern Kansas farm. I, too, loved riding on our old farm near a small central Kansas town called Partridge. I had also become somewhat attached to the ambiance and excitement of the horse track. In my time away from medical school, I had a job selling imported china and crystal primarily in New Mexico. On my days off I did all I could to spend time betting on quarter horse races in Raton or the beautiful hideaway called Ruidoso Downs. Between the Army's scholarship, my china sales, plus a little money from betting on the horses I was able to graduate from medical school with a little money in my pocket and not a penny in debt.

The day after I graduated, I packed all I owned including my doctor's bag, courtesy of Eli Lily who in those years gave one to every graduating medical student. Everything fit well into my 1952 green Hudson Hornet, and I was off to Louisville. Miriam came later. To this day, we cherish our days in Louisville (and the Derby) and can confirm that this book would likely not have been written if I had ended up in Saint Paul or Fort Worth for internship.

Training and studying at Louisville General Hospital was everything and more than we had hoped for. Trauma, addiction, infections, cancers. You name it. Louisville at the time was a poor city with lots of folks who needed charity medical care at a general hospital. What's more, the old Louisville General Hospital attracted some top-notch professors with big hearts. Out of the blue one day, my chief resident informed me that Dr. Robert Hoagland was coming to pay us a visit. My response was "Who is Dr. Hoagland?" With considerable reverence my chief said, "The Colonel is the world's expert on mononucleosis." My next question went something like this, "Did you say colonel?", "Well, yes.", "Is he in the Army?", "Yes.", "Why is he coming?" "Does he know I'm Army?"

To this day, I don't exactly know why the Colonel came to Louisville. Handsome and dressed in his peace-time uniform, he appeared in the Fall of 1966. He had just written his seminal book of 500 cases and was eager to teach not only me but all the other interns and residents. At the time I didn't think much about it, but he singled me out and we became great acquaintances. He was somehow aware that I would be joining him soon on active duty as a US Army Medical Officer. I learned a lot from this man who I came to consider the "old master," not just about IM, but what it meant to be a soldier and medical officer at the same time. He had committed himself to a lifetime US Army surgeon and officer career, and to being excellent in both roles. He left Louisville after a few days. During this time and in our later communications, he taught me about the intricacies of the disease, IM. At that time the Henles had not yet discovered that EBV caused IM. Dr. Hoagland, however, had already figured out that a virus had to be the cause of IM. He had unsuccessfully tried to treat IM with antibiotics and anti-fungal drugs. Since the disease did not respond to either of these agents, he correctly assumed that a virus had to be responsible for IM. He had learned from his 500 cases that corticosteroids knocked out IM in short shrift and prevented any serious complications. He started with 80 mg of prednisone on day one and tapered the dose downward over a few days. Out of 500 cases he never had a death or serious complication. He imbued me to treat soldiers who had IM with corticosteroids to keep them fit and combat ready. When I went active duty with the Army, I spent most of my time in Germany. Miriam and I lived in officers' quarters in Aschaffenburg, Wurzburg, and Heidelberg. All of our officer's living quarters were originally built by Hitler during World War II. I treated dozens of soldiers who had IM with the Hoagland protocol and never had a serious complication. I came to firmly believe that IM can almost always be well-controlled with corticosteroids, and I advocate them for use today with EBV R&A. Some physicians resist the use of corticosteroids in IM, but I believe low, intermittent use of corticosteroids are of great benefit in persons with EBV R&A mainly because they suppress glial cell activation and neuroinflammation.[39,53,59,62,96]

When Dr. Hoagland visited Louisville General, I had a case of a 19-year-old girl who had entered the hospital on October 2, 1966. She had IM and was quite ill and complained of bloody urine of three days duration. On her 20th hospital day, we did a kidney biopsy which showed non-streptococcal glomerulonephritis. The young woman eventually recovered, but both Dr. Hoagland and I believed her illness and hospitalization could have been prevented if she had received corticosteroids when her IM first started. I reported this case in the Texas Reports of Biology and Medicine in 1969.[101] Some other cases of glomerulonephritis with IM have subsequently been observed.[7]

At the time I reported the case of glomerulonephritis, we knew nothing about EBV R&A. Our model of thinking was based on the phenomenal work of Dr. Alvin Coburn. He discovered that the streptococcus bacteria caused scarlet fever, rheumatic fever, rheumatic heart disease, and glomerulonephritis. The initiating streptococcal infection was in the throat (strep throat), but the subsequent complications and diseases were distant in the body from the throat. The working theory was that the infectious agent either had to travel from the throat to the skin and heart or emit some toxic substance that traveled through the blood to the heart and kidneys. The knowledge that an infectious agent could form an antibody, called an autoantibody, that could attack tissues and cause disease, had not yet become common medical knowledge. Later in 1974, it was clearly known that IM produced autoantibodies.[94] As emphasized throughout this book, autoantibodies can form during IM or reactivated EBV and cause tissue destruction at any number of anatomic sites in the body.

In recent times several post IM complications have been observed. This includes rare cases of meningitis, hepatitis, pneumonia, and leg paralysis known as Guillain-Barre Syndrome. It is unclear if autoantibodies formed during acute IM continue to be active and if they are asymptomatic, but active, after resolution of acute IM. This is entirely possible since many persons who develop SCP and IP have had IM. A condition first described in 1988 and known as "chronic mononucleosis syndrome" or "chronic active Epstein-Barr infection" have been identified since the Hoagland book was published.[78,83,90] This is a severe, symptomatic disease. There is fever, painful throat, cervical adenopathy, and prostration resulting in a bed bound state. Severe symptomatic Epstein-Barr infection may also occur after organ transplants. Overwhelming infection may occasionally cause death. It is to be clearly noted that this book is dedicated only to EBV R&A which is a chronic asymptomatic disease that may result in cancer or a painful disease.

Each year two annual year books for disease treatment are published for the desktop of every physician: (1) Conn's Current Therapy, and (2) Current Medical Diagnosis and Treatment.[25,59] The 2024 editions essentially echo the treatments for acute infectious mononucleosis advocated by Dr. Hoagland in 1967. Both books acknowledge that IM may have rare sequelae such as meningitis, hepatitis, and glomerulonephritis. Both describe symptomatic chronic IM infection and the unfortunate situation when severe symptomatic IM develops after an organ transplant.

Only the 2024 Current Diagnosis and Treatment edition mentions that reactivation of EBV can occur. According to this source, reactivation only occurs in persons with a compromised or deficient immune system.[65] There is no mention that a major risk and hazard of EBV R&A is the potential development of cancer and intractable pain. It is important to point out that these two yearly excellent books are the bedrock of medical practice. They are essential for a top-notch medical practitioner. When a disease or condition is neither mentioned nor briefly described in these books, it is because the condition is uncommon or new. EBV R&A fits both of these situations and is a major reason this book has been written. EBV R&A is a newly recognized condition that hits persons who have an impaired immune system due to a chronic disease, genetic deficiency, or some stressful situation. For example, trauma, such as a fall or automobile accident can put a healthy person in jeopardy since their immune system is stressed and may allow EBV reactivation to silently begin.

Interestingly, I was indirectly involved in an IM complication that probably isn't well known outside the city of Louisville. The town in the last century was known in many places as the "town for boxers." Several champions came out of Louisville including Mohammed Ali (Cassius Clay). The Golden Gloves were a "big thing" in Louisville. I volunteered to do pre-fight physicals on Louisville Golden Glove boxers. Dr. Hoagland had a simple message. Always check for an enlarged spleen because it may stay enlarged for months after IM has resolved.[46] There were rumors that some spleens had ruptured during active boxing matches and that a couple of boxers had died from the incident. Indeed, I and my fellow doctors who did the pre-fight physicals stopped a few kids from entering the ring due to a large spleen. Needless to say, we weren't always popular with all the boxers around the Golden Glove culture in Louisville.

The Epstein-Barr Virus:

My wife and I left Louisville in 1967 and headed for Galveston, Texas. The Army gave me another year to study as a resident at the University of Texas Medical Branch where they treated a lot of tuberculosis and tropical, infectious diseases. During my year, I took preceptorship opportunities to study rare infectious diseases at the New Orleans General Hospital and spent some time at the Carville, Louisiana leper colony. Leprosy was a horrible, slow-moving infection in those days. It is now well-controlled with antibiotics. The colony is now the National Leprosarium Museum. I was well prepared for my first assignment on active Army duty which was to care for the soldiers in Vietnam who had tropical infectious diseases and were Med-E-Vaced to Brooke Army Hospital in San Antonio, Texas. By the time I started active duty with the Army in late 1968, I had learned one thing about infections. They can cause weird, unpredictable diseases. The fact that EBV can reactivate, create autoimmunity, and produce terrible diseases, is not a surprise.

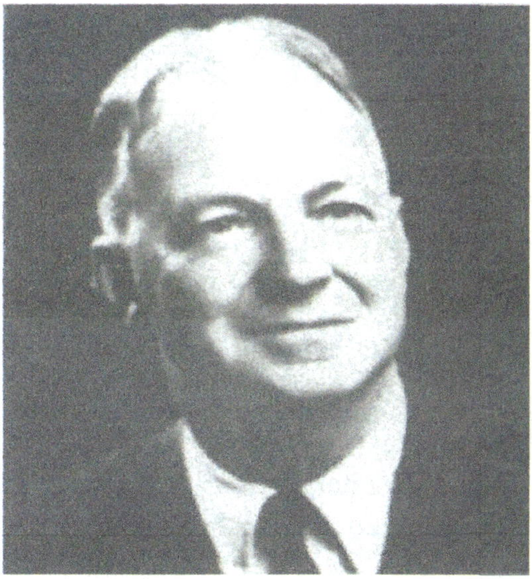

Alvin F. Coburn, MD discovered that streptococcal throat infections may cause scarlet fever, rheumatic fever, rheumatic heart disease, and glomerulonephritis after the acute infection has subsided. This was the first documented evidence that an infection could cause an autoimmune process that leads to diseases after the acute infection has resolved. These diseases were initially called "collagen diseases." EBV causes infectious mononucleosis, and, after it is resolved, some diseases may result due to an autoimmune process.

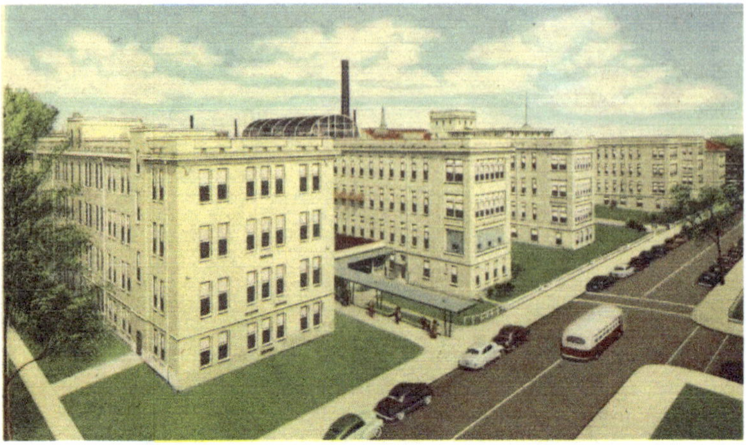

Louisville General Hospital, Louisville, Kentucky (circa 1965).

7. A Great Discovery: EBV Reactivation

After Dr. Epstein convinced Werner and Gertrude Henle to validate his findings that a virus caused a cancer, it didn't take them long to duplicate his monumental discovery. The Henles were brilliant workaholics who loved their work. They not only verified the findings of Drs. Epstein and Barr but quickly realized that the virus was a transmissible infection that could cause cancers and IM. They were unaware that EBV could cause painful diseases.

Since EBV was a transmitted infection, the Henles correctly assumed that the human body tried to resist or fight off the virus by forming antibodies which are the body's main weapon to fight off infections. In a relatively short time, the Henles and their first-class team of associates determined that the body formed antibodies to ward off EBV, and they developed the antibody tests for EBV that are still used today.[40,41] The first major antibody they found was against the viral capsule or capsid now labeled as VCA (viral capsule antibody). A second antibody was formed against the interior or nucleus of the virus now called EBNA (Epstein-Barr nuclear antibody).

After developing the antibody tests, the Henle team found that the children who had Burkitt's tumors had extremely high levels of EBV antibodies.[41] The importance of developing antibody tests was that they are a measuring tool to see if EBV may be the cause of a disease. The Henle teamed up with some other topflight researchers to initially test patients with sarcoidosis and some forms of lymphoma and leukemia to see if EBV caused these diseases.[44,66] The EBV antibody levels were inconclusive in these diseases. The antibody tests weren't questionable, however, when in 1970, they tested patients with Hodgkin's disease, which is a lymph node cancer. The EBV antibody levels matched the high levels found in Burkitt's lymphoma.[42,56,57] Dr. Harold Von Hanson in his most descriptive biography of the Henle work, stated that Werner Henle believed the high EBV antibodies found in Hodgkin's disease were a result of EBV reactivation. In other words, the patients with Hodgkin's had EBV active in their bodies but didn't know anything was wrong until they woke up one day with cancer.

Unfortunately, reactivation and autoimmunity of EBV is a silent, asymptomatic process in which the unsuspecting person isn't aware until cancer or a painful disease becomes apparent. Even today the concept of EBV reactivation is largely unknown, but the fact is that EBV can reactivate and silently produce cancers and painful diseases with no overt symptoms to alert the person that "something is wrong" until the disease is well-advanced.

To prove that reactivation may occur the Henles teamed up with an infectious disease specialist and epidemiologist named Dr. Ciro Valent Sumaya.[91,92] They took blood samples from 962 individuals in 109 households in a rural area of Louisiana. Out of this group they found that 20 adults had sky high antibody tests which they believed had to be due to reactivation of EBV. The results of the Louisiana study were published in two papers entitled:

1. Seroepidemiologic Study of Epstein-Barr Virus Infections in a Rural Community;[91]

2. Endogenous Reactivation of Epstein-Barr Virus Infections.[92]

These studies made two specific points. First, they showed that reactivation may be totally asymptomatic. Second, they were able to determine that EBV reactivation isn't very common although over 95% of the adult population has been exposed to EBV and are carriers of the virus.

EBV antibody testing has been used to determine if reactivation may be a causative factor in a number of diseases including rheumatoid arthritis, systemic lupus, Sjogren's syndrome, multiple sclerosis, and some cancers. EBV reactivation is now accepted to play a role in some lymphomas, Hodgkin's disease, nasopharyngeal and gastric cancers.[103] Some estimates are that EBV is now responsible for at least 2% of the world's cancers.

After some minor technical alterations, the Henle antibody tests were put into commercial use in the last part of the 1900's. These antibody tests now make it possible for any medical practitioner to determine if a patient has reactivated EBV and likely has autoimmunity. In a later chapter, I report the results of my study of 110 patients with IP due to adhesive arachnoiditis (AA). Also, I give my recommendations on correlating EBV antibody tests to clinical manifestations in order to make a presumptive diagnosis of EBV R&A. A major characteristic initially identified by Drs. Henle and Sumaya is that EBV reactivation is a silent process that is ongoing until it results in cancer or a painful disease.

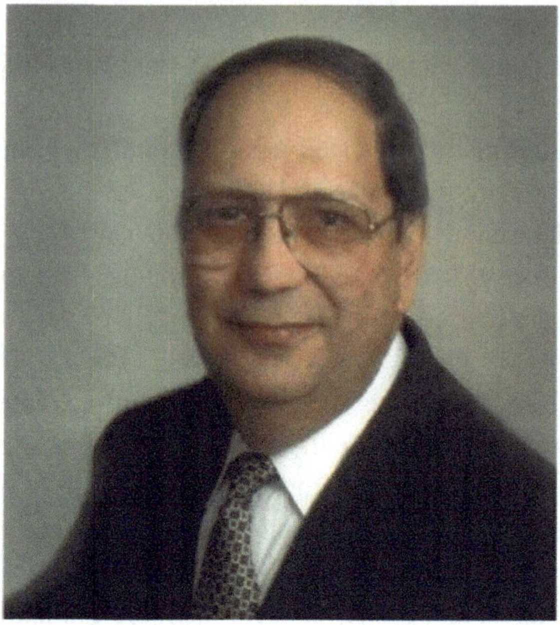

Ciro Valent Sumaya, MD worked with Drs. Werner and Gertrude Henle to test persons for EBV antibodies in a rural Louisiana community. It was found that some persons had EBV reactivation. Dr. Sumaya was the first to publish that EBV infection can reactivate. His seminal report in 1977 was entitled, "Endogenous Reactivation of Epstein-Barr Virus Infection."

8. How EBV Reactivation Causes Chronic and Intractable Pain

The definition of EBV reactivation is a "change from a dormant, carrier state to one in which the virus begins to duplicate and becomes an active infectious agent that can produce painful diseases and cancer."

EBV can reactivate from its normal latent state under stress conditions.[26,28,61,65] The stress that can cause reactivation can be trauma, infection, malnutrition, fatigue, and even psychological. In this sense, the virus is "opportunistic" in that the latent virus takes an opportunity to reactivate and begin to replicate (duplicate) because the stress has hampered one's natural immune system. This is called the "lytic" phase. Lymphocytes infected with reactivated EBV may carry the virus through the blood stream and enter any number of tissues including the central nervous system (brain and spinal cord). In this manner the virus may infiltrate tissues. A lymphocyte that carries reactivated EBV may become a plasma cell and develop autoantibodies.[71]

The major characteristic of reactivation is that it may not produce symptoms over a long time period. Unfortunately, reactivation can cause cancer or painful disease before the person is aware that a serious pathologic event has been taking place inside their body. In this regard, EBV reactivation is like diabetes. One may have an elevated blood sugar that has initiated a disease process, but the person never knows about it until a blood vessel clogs up and causes a leg ulcer or heart attack. A major goal of this book is to educate persons to test and identify EBV R&A as soon as possible so it can be controlled and contained before serious disease sets in.

Reactivation episodes are variable in length and intensity. Although precise details are unknown, a reactivation episode may last days to years. The length and intensity can be influenced by the stress that caused the reactivation. Once the stress is over, such as an infection or traumatic injury, the body's natural immune system may suppress the reactivation and return the EBV to its natural dormant, harmless, carrier state. Once antibodies and autoantibodies are formed, however, they may remain elevated and active for life. A person may have several reactivation periods in a lifetime. A person who has an innate compromised immune system such as is found in genetic connective tissue or autoimmune diseases are more prone to EBV reactivation and autoimmunity.[74] An infection by bacteria such as Lyme or mycoplasma and viruses including cytomegalovirus, rubella, herpes six, and covid may amplify or accelerate reactivation.

Today, almost all clinical laboratories offer EBV antibody tests that show a normal range so elevated levels of the two major antibodies that indicate reactivation can be evaluated. They are viral capsid (capsule) antibody which is abbreviated VCA and the other is known as viral nuclear antibody and abbreviated as EBNA. High levels above normal range indicate that reactivation has taken place in the past and/or is currently present. Extremely high levels suggest that the patient has either had a single severe reactivation or more likely had multiple reactivations over time. A relatively new test called early nuclear antigen antibody (early EBNA) is indicative of current active reactivation and is a signal to start aggressive medical measures to control the virus.

Once EBV is reactivated it may cause a painful disease by three possible different pathologic mechanisms.

#1- Tissue Infiltration

One look at the children pictured on the cover of this book and there should be no doubt that EBV can infiltrate tissues and cause disease. Lymphocytes that carry EBV in the blood stream may enter any tissue in the body. Once the infected lymphocyte enters a tissue site, it may release EBV into the tissue where it may flourish and replicate.

#2- Toxic Substances

All living cells including EBV contain deoxyribonucleic acid (DNA) as a component. The cells, therefore, will excrete waste products which may be toxic. Although no specific EBV toxin has been identified, it is theorized by many observers that the virus emits one or more toxic substances. Some believe that the viral capsule that is left behind as a residue in tissues when the virus replicates is toxic.

#3- Autoimmunity

It has been traditional since the 1940's that a disease is labeled as autoimmune when it is associated with an autoantibody. The definition of autoantibody is a globulin that attacks normal tissue to cause inflammation, tissue destruction, scarring, and pain. Lymphocytes that carry reactivated EBV may become plasma cells and produce autoantibodies that are part of the nuclear antibody, EBNA. Also, some researchers believe that reactivated EBV may attack and cross-react with normal tissue to produce an autoimmune process within the tissues.

It has been known for several years that some autoimmune diseases such as rheumatoid arthritis and systemic lupus are, as a group, associated with high EBV antibody levels.[3,11,22,47,73,105,110] There has been debate ("and resistance?") to the idea that a single virus could be responsible for so many diseases.[38] In a later chapter, I present our EBV antibody findings in adhesive arachnoiditis (AA). Our findings appear quite clear and convincing. The difference in the two situations is that AA is preceded by one or more obvious conditions or risk factors such as an inherited connective tissue disease such as Ehlers-Danlos syndrome or spine trauma. EBV R&A functions as an intermediate or catalytic step in the development of AA. In the classic autoimmune diseases such as rheumatoid arthritis, there are no clearly identified precondition or risk factors so the notion that EBV is the sole cause of the disease is justifiably controversial. The recent research by Dr. John Harley and associates may resolve the controversy. The Harley studies indicate that EBV can trigger the genes of several diseases including rheumatoid arthritis and multiple sclerosis which, in contrast to AA, don't have clear preconditions or risk factors.

It is now clear that most, if not all, cases of SCP and IP have a preexisting condition or risk factor that makes the individual a prime candidate for the development of EBV R&A. In the attached schemata, there is a list of stressful conditions that may reactivate latent and dormant EBV and create a detrimental pathologic pathway.

In summary, EBV reactivation mainly occurs in persons with an impaired immunity that may be a component of a genetic disease, autoimmune disease, or temporary stressful situation. EBV reactivation produces an autoimmune disorder with autoantibodies. A person may undergo multiple, periodic reactivation episodes. Unfortunately, EBV R&A is initially asymptomatic so the person with it is unaware that a serious pathologic consequence such as IP may be underway.

TABLE

THREE CHARACTERISTICS OF
EBV REACTIVATION AND AUTOIMMUNITY

- ✓ Silent and asymptomatic until a painful condition or cancer develops
- ✓ Occurs primarily in persons with a compromised immune system
- ✓ A person may have multiple reactivations throughout life
- ✓ The stress that causes reactivation may be trauma, stroke, infection, nutritional, fatigue, or psychologic

HOW EBV REACTIVATION CAUSES SEVERE CHRONIC AND INTRACTABLE PAIN

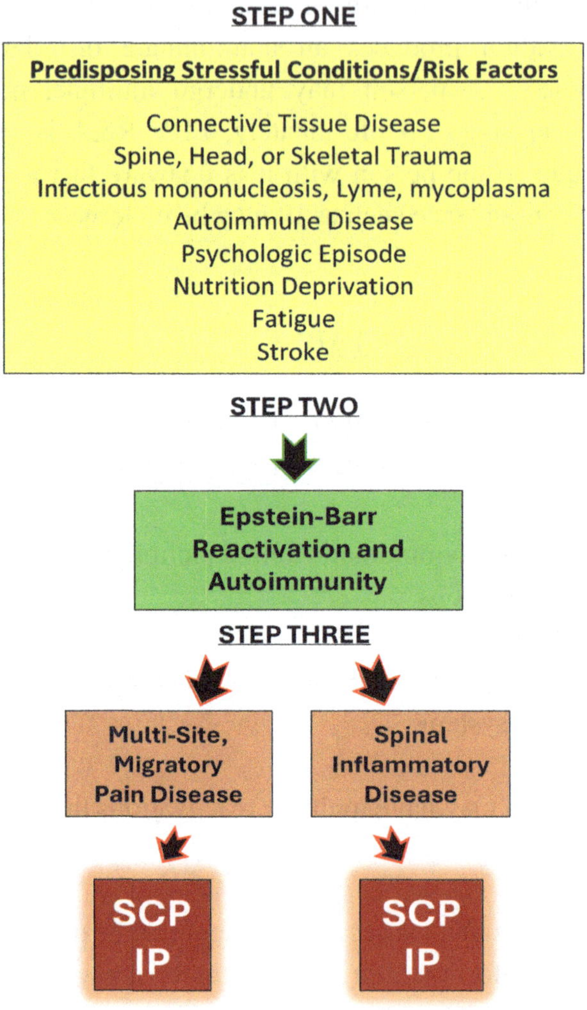

There may be stressful conditions other than those listed here that initiate EBV R&A or intractable pain. EBV reactivation and autoimmunity fundamentally act as a catalyst in the development of severe chronic and intractable pain.

9. The Bane of Intractable Pain

Chronic pain (CP) is usually defined as a pain that persists longer than the usual healing time of 90 days.[32,80,99] Within the group of chronic pain patients are two subgroups. One is "severe, chronic pain" (SCP) which is about 10% and the other is "intractable pain" (IP) which is about 2% of the chronic pain population. SCP and IP differ from run-of-the-mill chronic pain in that these individuals require daily analgesic medication for relief. Consequently, these two subgroups constitute the great majority of pain patients who need regular care from medical practitioners. Persons with IP differ from SCP in that they have constant, incurable pain that produces cardiovascular, respiratory, endocrine, and metabolic complications.[99] Most medical practitioners don't differentiate between SCP and IP which is perfectly acceptable from the viewpoint of medical treatment.

IP has plagued and befuddled medical practitioners for centuries. This subgroup of chronic pain patients has been variously labeled. In recent times, such labels as persistent, central, neuropathic, or high impact have been used. The term intractable has emerged in the United States as the most common term for the severe, chronic, incurable pain patient.[99] Many states now have IP laws that give medical practitioners authority to prescribe opioids and other potent medicinals to these tragic individuals. There are two longstanding overriding questions which involve SCP and IP regardless of any label that has been applied. One is why two patients with seemingly the same degree of injury or disease have greatly different pain levels. The other is why some chronic pain patients develop SCP or IP while the usual chronic pain patient has rather simple, intermittent or periodic episodes of mild or moderate pain that varies in severity, intensity, and responds to a wide variety of therapeutic measures such as anti-inflammatory agents, topical skin applications, physical measures, and electromedical devices.

Dr. John Fothergill was the most famous physician of the 18th century. He summarized today's perplexity about SCP and IP relative to its complexity, causation, confusion, and reluctance of physicians to treat it. In his 1781 book entitled "A Complete Collection of the Medical Philosophical Work of John Fothergill, MD" he stated,

> *"The name rheumatism-or, as it is now more precisely termed, chronic rheumatism-has been used as a generic term for persistent pains, unaccompanied by constitutional disturbance, irrespective of their causation, and has covered an unknown amount of carelessness and ignorance; while, as a verbal placebo, it has often been used to justify a do-nothing treatment, sometimes very reprehensible."*
> (Pater-Nofter-Row, London, p684-686)

It is most interesting that Dr. Fothergill referred to what I now call "multi-site migratory pain disease" which is described in detail in the next chapter. He said a property of "rheumatism" is, "it has rapid metastases, of suddenly quitting one part to manifest itself in another; on other occasions it lingers around one part with great pertinacity."

Based on my studies and observations, Dr. Fothergill was probably encountering EBV multi-site migratory pain typical of EBV R&A.

In the latter part of the 20th century patients with IP tended to have a straight-forward "cause and effect." Patients had a single cause of pain such as post-herpetic neuralgia, trauma, systemic lupus, arteriosclerosis, chronic pancreatitis, abdominal adhesions, or rheumatoid arthritis. The severe back pain patient was often labeled as "failed back surgery syndrome" because they had undergone spine surgery, but the pain didn't resolve.

Fortunately, many medical advances and specific treatments have emerged in recent years to ameliorate several SCP and IP conditions that were common in the last century. This welcome advent has reduced the need to provide potent and risky pain treatments for many patients who formerly required such measures as high dose opioids and implanted electrical stimulators. Notable examples are specific pharmacologic agents for interstitial cystitis, autoimmune diseases, sickle cell anemia, and herpes zoster. In addition, metallic implants for severe osteoarthritis of the hip and knee joints have markedly reduced severe pain in many individuals. New treatments for arteriosclerosis and diabetes have reduced the degree of pain related to neuropathies and arthropathies caused by these conditions.

Due to the many medical advances in the last part of the 20th century, the underlying causes that motivated patients to seek pain treatment began to change in the 1990's. Patients who resembled Dr. Fothergill's description of persistent migratory pain began to seek relief and, in my experience, constitute most of today's patients who have SCP and IP. The next chapter describes what I term "Multi-site, Migratory Pain Disease."

Literally for centuries, physicians have wondered why some patients and not others develop SCP and IP. A brilliant neurologic scientist, Dr. Linda Watkins, around the turn of the century found that glial cells in the brain and spinal cord were activated by pain.[111,112] When over-activated the cells produced neuroinflammation that destroyed tissue in the brain and spinal cord. Her work was confirmed in 2004 when Dr. Vania Apkarian and his research team found, by use of special brain scans, that persons with chronic back pain reduced the gray matter in brain tissues.[6]

These two groundbreaking findings have now been duplicated and confirmed by multiple research groups.[17,21,23,69,70,76,84] The significance of these scientific discoveries has finally provided an explanation for the question as to why some patients, but not others, develop SCP and IP. Many persons who develop SCP and IP have a loss of brain tissue due to glial cell activation and neuroinflammation.[87,102,106] Brain tissue contains biochemicals known as neurotransmitters that activate or stimulate action points known as receptors to stop pain. Obviously, if brain tissue is anatomically deficient, the neurotransmitters and receptors that normally put a stop to pain, aren't available.[113,116] The poor person afflicted is, therefore, left in constant pain.

Although first class science in this century has told us that anatomical loss of brain and spinal cord tissue may result in constant SCP or IP, the reason that glial cells activate and produce neuroinflammation has been unclear. I mention in the introduction of this book that new research has shown that EBV can cause glial cell activation and neuroinflammation.[50,51,52]

There may be other viruses or causes of glial cell activation, but EBV is now clearly known to be a cause.[1] This is a major reason why EBV is now a factor in chronic pain care.

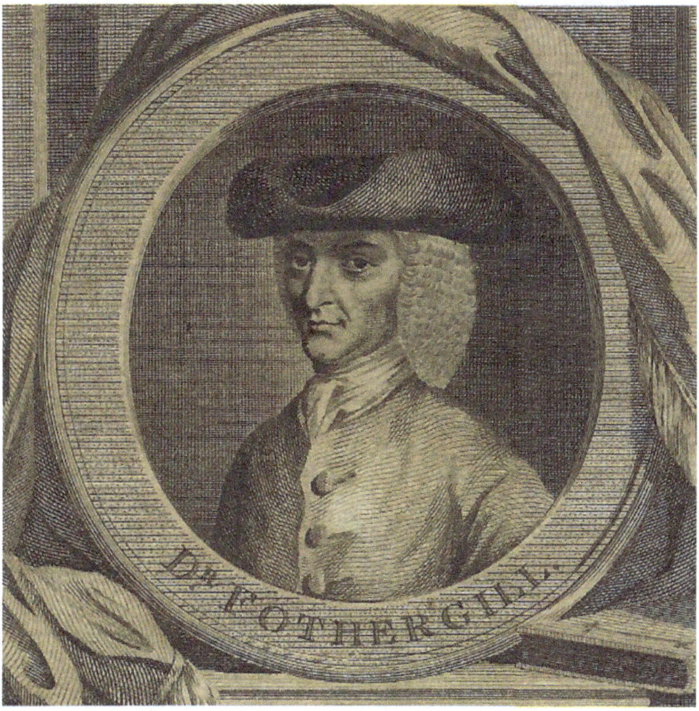

Dr. John Fothergill was the most famous British physician in the 1700's. He called chronic or intractable pain, rheumatism. He observed that some patients had pain in one anatomic site, but it would migrate to another. He felt the patient must have some sort of "blood poison."

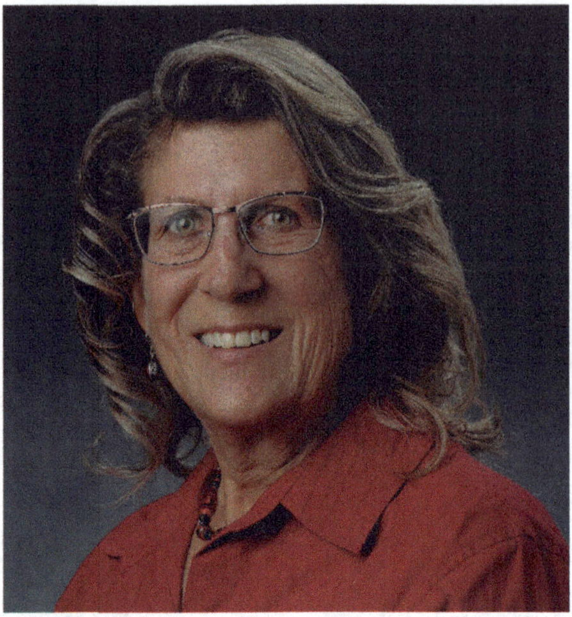

Linda Watkins, PhD, was the first to recognize that glial cells would activate and create neuroinflammation that led to intractable pain.

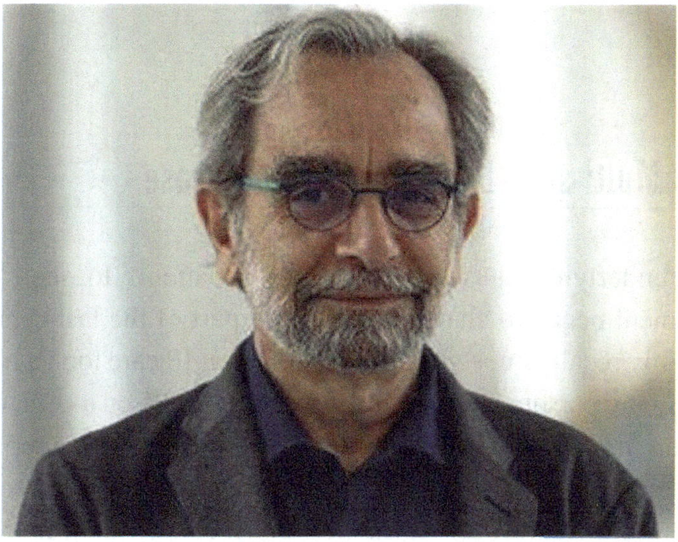

Dr. Vania Apkarian was the first to show by brain scan that severe chronic pain causes a loss of gray matter in the brain.

10. Multi-site, Migratory Pain Disease

The underlying causes that prompted patients to seek pain treatment began to change in the latter part of the last century. I vividly recall almost the day and hour that IP care took a major turn in my personal care of patients. It was 1995 on a cool, crisp Spring day in West Covina. A retired schoolteacher was referred to me by a physician who said, "she needs narcotics, but I can't figure out what's wrong with her." My IP clinic which I started in 1975, treated uncommon pain patients who were referred by their physicians. The clinic operated a few days a month and was fundamentally a clinic in which patients could essentially pay what they could afford. Criteria for referral of IP patients was failure of standard pain treatments and a need for palliative care to prevent premature death. Families had to attend with the patients. The clinic never had over 100 enrollees as many reached terminus or were placed with another physician.

I noticed the lady in the waiting room. She was nicely dressed, didn't appear disabled or sick, and showed the kindly manner of a retired teacher in her sixties. This alone was a surprise. Most patients with IP who needed narcotics, now called opioids, had tell-tale signs of IP such as frailty, a paralytic limb, prosthesis, wheelchair, or colorless skin. Between 1975 and 1995 the underlying causes of IP were rather obvious and included metastatic cancer, neurologic impairments from trauma, or a rheumatologic disease. Above all, they looked and were quite ill. Not so, with the lady I was about to evaluate.

My usual first question was always, "What and why do you have pain." Her answers were "fibromyalgia" and "I hurt all over." My physical examination only showed some possible tenderness around her chest and ankles. Reflexes, muscle strength, and neurologic function were all within normal limits. I was perplexed when she said she needed the equivalent of about 200 mg of morphine a day to stay comfortable. I was even more perplexed when I asked when and how her pain started. She stated, "I don't know. I just woke up about six months ago and had so much pain (all over) I couldn't get out of bed."

Until this lady showed up, anyone who came to our clinic and didn't show a clear cause of pain and requested opioids was considered a drug addict. They always, however, looked the part. Not this lady. She didn't smoke, drink, have tattoos or drive a half-wrecked jalopy. She was a refined, normal person and not a member of the drug-seeking crowd around Los Angeles who were easily recognized at a glance. Furthermore, she had a daughter with her who vouched for her veracity.

My next step with the woman was to rule out psychiatric disease and to run some laboratory tests. I had her fill out some handy screening tests for anxiety and depression that were tools developed by an innovative psychiatrist named Aaron Beck. I also gave her a lengthy psychiatric test called the Multi-Minnesota Personality Inventory (MMPI). She proved to have all her mental faculties and was nowhere near being a psycho.

My laboratory evaluation included a complete blood count, inflammatory markers, and immunologic tests for rheumatoid arthritis and systemic lupus. The tests showed some minor changes in her serum proteins and white blood cell count which were just enough to convince me that the patient had a real problem. I chose to keep her as a patient in our IP clinic that consisted of some 50 attendees at the time of which many were near terminus. She looked out-of-place since she wasn't terminal, but I wanted to learn more about what I considered to be a "new but bothersome experience."

At the time this woman became my patient, I was aware of fibromyalgia but questioned whether it was a real disease or just another Hollywood fad. My inquiries to physicians that I highly respected informed me that fibromyalgia was a legitimate disease, but its causes were unknown and there was no treatment for it.

At her second clinic visit, about 10-14 days after her first, she came with an ace wrap on her wrist. She said she had carpal tunnel syndrome. Also, she had been having some migraine headaches. At the time, I thought they were unconnected, unrelated events. Over the next few months, however, it seemed like she had a new complaint each visit. One month it was burning feet, and another irritable bowel or back pain. Also, another of her doctors told her she had hypothyroidism and had started her on thyroid medication. Interestingly, her carpal tunnel resolved, and her headaches and muscle pains seemed to get better, but her back pain got worse. Regardless, she always complained of "pain all over."

Within a few months I received another referral with "pain all over." Then came a third and fourth. All had fibromyalgia and pain in a multitude of anatomic locations. I began to believe "something new must be happening" in the general population. It felt like the spread of an infectious epidemic as in flu season.

I hadn't seen these kinds of cases, and they appeared over a relatively short time period. The patients made me uncomfortable because I couldn't initially discern any physical signs of disease that were typical in the usual IP patient. To get to the bottom of this new development, I started to examine these patients in a more detailed manner. Sure enough, I found subtle signs of physical abnormalities when they tried to wrinkle their brow, flex their ankles, or stand up straight. Their back muscles showed asymmetry and even areas of muscle contracture and indentation. Also, many had minor changes in white blood counts, serum proteins, and inflammatory markers. Both physical and laboratory signs were minor, but they provided some legitimacy for the "pain all over" cases.

Within a couple of years after I had accepted the "pain all over" retired teacher, I had about two dozen similar cases. The referring doctors usually had no idea what caused the pain, but the patient required opioids and sometimes couldn't get out of bed without them. Patients had good families and usually didn't smoke or drink heavily. Most gave a history that they literally woke up one morning with "pain all over." Complaints included back, arm, thigh, and headache pain, and patients were frustrated because the pain seemed to migrate from one site to another. All had been given the new popular diagnosis of fibromyalgia even though pain didn't always include muscles.

I tried to get some opinions and insight into these patients from other physicians including pain specialists. No doctor I consulted had any answer except they thought fibromyalgia was probably real. In recent years brain scans studies show a loss of gray matter in the brains of fibromyalgia and "pain all over" cases.[8,86] The brain tissue loss seems to follow rather than precede the onset of pain. Also, it is now well-recognized that fibromyalgia is associated with other painful conditions.[16,97,98]

By the year 2000, I believed that one or more virus infections were the basic cause of at least some cases of "pain all over." My reason was simply that something had to cause pain in multiple sites and then migrate to new ones. I recalled not only Dr. Fothergill's description of "rheumatism" but the physicians in the 1800's who believed in what they called "autoinfection." This meant that a parasite, usually a bacterium in the intestine, would travel through the bloodstream and cause different organs and tissues to become painful and diseased. The 1900 Gould and Pyle Cyclopedia of Medicine and Surgery" provides great detail about the symptoms and recommended treatment for autoinfection.[36] Of keen interest is that autoinfection could cause pain due to polymyositis which is pain in multiple muscles. Today this condition is often called "myofascial syndrome."

I had a motivating moment when I learned that my first fibromyalgia "pain all over" patient, the retired schoolteacher, had deteriorated and became bed bound. She died about six years after her first visit to my office. My thought was that she had some progressive and unknown infectious or metabolic disease. Her death motivated me to pursue my hunch that a virus or viruses were responsible.

Migration of pain sites compelled me to believe that only a virus could travel through the blood to multiple sites. Autoimmunity was also a consideration. It didn't dawn on me at the time that both tissue infiltration and autoimmunity could simultaneously operate and even be caused by the same virus. Given my viral theory in the first decade of this century, I began to take viral blood tests on almost all my IP patients. Some of the tests were imperfect as only titers rather than serum levels were available in the laboratories. A numerical or quantitative serum level usually means that you have a cut off between normal and abnormal which is what is needed for topnotch research. Titers are less specific. Nevertheless, I could obtain either titers or numerical level values for not only EBV but varicella, rubella, coxsackie, herpes, and cytomegalovirus. If I thought the patient had multiple anatomic pain sites that migrated, I began to administer one of three antiviral agents: (1) acyclovir (Zovirax®), (2) valacyclovir (Valtrex®), or (3) famciclovir (Famvir®).

Most, but not all, patients seemed to reduce their pain. My blood test results were, admittedly, quite confusing to me. Almost all patients had two or more positive titers or elevated quantitative levels of antibodies. My initial thoughts were that it must be a combination of two or more viruses that caused multi-site, migratory pain. My thoughts now are that there is a "primary" or "lead" virus and others seem to follow or be "secondary." Usually, but not always, EBV is the lead.

Over the next few years, I continued viral testing and treatment and wrote and presented two abstracts on my viral work at medical meetings. These meetings today have their standard oral presentations, but new and early scientific research is presented as a research poster or in a book of abstracts given to all attendees. In this manner, physicians and scientists interested in new, hopefully breakthrough, studies can discuss the finding with the investigator. My two abstracts were presented at multiple meetings including the American Pain Society, American Academy of Pain Medicine, and American Academy of Pain Management.

One study was called "Does Viral Suppression Therapy Enhance Pain Control in Selected Fibromyalgia Patients" and the other was "Viral Titers in Sudden-Onset Chronic Pain Disorders." Both of the abstracts are presented here verbatim primarily for historic documentation and to give all parties my early thoughts and experiences with viruses and pain.

Abstract Presented in 2010 at the American Academy of Pain Management

Does Viral suppression Therapy Enhance Pain Control in Selected Fibromyalgia Patients?

Forest Tennant M.D., Dr. P.H., Laura Herman RN, NP Veract Research Clinic, West Covina, CA.

Introduction: Some cases of fibromyalgia demonstrate severe, persistent pain which is difficult to control even with high dosages of opioid drugs. To date there is neither standard therapy for fibromyalgia nor accepted causation, although viral infection has been postulated as a possible cause of some cases.

Materials and Methods: Seven fibromyalgia patients who had experienced numerous symptomatic treatments and were maintained with opioids at 400 - 1000mg/dl of morphine equivalence were studied. Pain control was judged to be poor to fair. Subjects demonstrated positive serum titers at least two times normal to two of more of the following viral agents: (1) cytomegalus; (2) rubella; (3) varicella, (4) herpes simplex; (5) Epstein Barr. Titers indicated either previous or possibly current infection. Patients were treated with either acyclovir,

400 to 1000mg/d, or valacyclovir, 500 to 1000mg/d. After one month patients were evaluated for pain reduction, endurance, well-being, and side-effects. If improved pain control was reported, viral suppression was indefinitely continued.

Results: All patients reported improvement in pain control, endurance, energy, and well-being. Two reported decrease in cervical lymph node size. Discontinuation of viral suppression for one week in three patients resulted in a resurgence of pain and other symptoms.

Conclusions: This preliminary study suggests that fibromyalgia patients with severe persistent pain and positive viral titers may experience enhanced pain control with viral suppression therapy. It also suggests that there is some unclear neuro-mechanism by which a previous or current viral infection may produce pain.

<u>Abstract Presented in 2014 at the American Pain society</u>

Can Viral Infections Cause Sudden-Onset of Intractable Pain?

Forest Tennant M.D., Dr.P.H., Veract Intractable Pain Clinic, West Covina, CA.

Introduction: Pain associated with human immunodeficiency virus (HIV), polio, hepatitis C, and herpes zoster is well known, so it is likely that other viruses may precipitate pain.

Objective: Determine if there is objective evidence that a viral infection may cause sudden, intractable pain. There are some intractable pain patients whose condition appeared suddenly, without warning, and with no apparent pre-disposing condition.

Methods: Six adult (three male and three female) intractable pain patients who suddenly developed their condition without warning or precipitating event were tested for these viral titers: Epstein-Barr, varicella, rubella, rubeola, cytomegalus, herpes I & II, and coxsackie. All patients recalled the precise day and date their intractable pain began and remained persistent despite multiple pain treatment measures. Two had onset of constant headaches, one had pelvic pain, and three had upper torso, myofascial pain. All six patients had two or more viral titers which were 5 to 40 times above the normal range. The high titers were Epstein-Barr, varicella, cytomegalus, or rubella viruses.

Comments: The mechanism of sudden persistent pain following a viral infection is unclear. Possible mechanisms include on-going viral activity, microglial cell activation and centralized pain, and the initiation of a systemic autoimmune disorder.

Summary: It is unknown if the initiating virus is still active in the patients studied here. The extremely high viral titers found in these patients who had a sudden onset of intractable pain are compatible with the notion that a viral infection may cause intractable pain.

After presentation of the abstracts above I continued to administer anti-viral drugs to IP patients. Although I did not do a controlled study, most patients claimed that anti-viral medication reduced their pain and their need for daily pain relief medications. My study goal was to determine the most common viruses which caused pain, and which antiviral agents and dosages were optimal. I concluded that some viruses must play a causative role in the development of multi-site, migratory pain. My top viral candidates for this honor were Epstein-Barr, cytomegalovirus, and rubella. All three are known to reactivate, and they seemed to be predominant in my pilot studies.[89,105] In addition, I believed that a virus or viruses were responsible for the transition from intermittent, mild, chronic pain to constant, severe IP.

I regularly heard from patients that multi-site, migratory pain preceded their IP condition which was primarily complex regional pain syndrome or adhesive arachnoiditis. Also, I had almost two dozen patients who had either sustained head trauma or a stroke and afterwards developed multi-site, migratory pain.[54] To determine if multi-site, migratory pain preceded a serious, IP condition, I surveyed 36 persons with AA who had high blood levels of EBV antibodies indicative of past and/or current reactivation. These persons were asked which painful conditions they experienced prior to developing AA. Their responses are in the attached table.

In summary, clinical reports from as long ago as the 1700s describe an entity that is properly called "multi-site, migratory pain disease." In my research, a majority of persons I encounter with SCP or IP started with multi-site, migratory pain disease and later developed a singular condition that caused the majority, but not all, of their pain. The end-stage condition in most of them has been lumbar or cervical neck pain.

TABLE

Painful Conditions That Preceded Adhesive Arachnoiditis in Patients With Elevated EBV Antibodies N = 36		
CONDITION	No.	%
Arthritis	36	100
Neuropathies	36	100
Herniated discs	29	80.5
Migraine	27	75
Fibromyalgia	22	61.1
Irritable bowel	21	58.3
Temporal mandibular joint (TMJ)	20	55.6
Tarlov cyst	18	50.0
Bursitis	18	50.0
Sciatica	17	47.2
Loss of teeth	17	47.2
Spinal fluid leaks	15	41.7
Plantar fasciitis	15	41.7
Tendonitis	13	36.1
Complex regional pain syndrome (CRPS)	9	25.0
Costochondritis	8	22.2

Persons in this study reported more than one condition. Also, the condition may have receded or continued after the development of adhesive arachnoiditis.

11. Spinal Inflammatory Disease

In the previous chapter, I called for labeling the person with multiple pain sites that vary over time, "Multi-Site, Migratory Pain Disease." Low back and neck pain are often sites of pain in a person with "multi-site, migratory pain disease" and very often the neck or lower back pain are the "end-stage" conditions which force the patient to seek medical help. Back pain has traditionally been the major cause of SCP and IP that brings a patient to a medical practitioner.

In this century there has been a concerted effort to identify specific disease entities that cause back pain. For example, as difficult as it is to believe, modern medicine has a diagnosis called "failed back surgery syndrome." Patients were operated on, but the pain didn't resolve, and their doctor didn't know why, so they gave "failure" a diagnosis. The fact is that medical practice didn't have enough tools to diagnose specific back ailments until this century, so they often did surgery hoping for the best. Contrast magnetic resonance imaging (MRI) has changed this situation. MRIs can visually separate spinal fluid from solid tissues in the spine so abnormalities can be spotted. Tissues that are inflamed including intervertebral discs, spinal canal cover (dura and arachnoid), vertebrae, and cauda equina nerves can all be visualized by the new MRI technology.[29,95,114] Thanks to this new technology, I have found inflammation in multiple spinal tissues that produce SCP or IP.

The Epstein-Barr Virus:

New laboratory tests help diagnose the presence of inflammation in various spinal tissues. Inflammatory markers called interleukins or cytokines have been developed and they have shown that inflammation is in degenerated herniated discs, spinal ligaments (e.g., ligamentum flavum), and in adhesive arachnoiditis.[9,29,63,95,114] In this chapter, a Table lists spinal conditions that may contribute to SCP and IP due to inflammation. The Table is a summary of 36 consecutive patients with MRI documented AA who were surveyed and asked what other spinal diseases they had when their diagnosis of AA was made. Adhesive arachnoiditis (AA) is a serious and tragic disease in which both the arachnoid membrane (inner lining of the spinal canal cover) and cauda equina nerves become inflamed, form adhesions, and glue together to form a nerve entrapment mass inside the spinal canal.[2,4,9] In the Tennant Foundation AA Research and Education Project, we have reviewed over 1200 MRIs from patients with AA. In every case there has been MRI evidence of inflammation in spinal tissues other than the cauda equina and arachnoid membrane. For example, almost every patient we have reviewed with AA has degenerated, protruding intervertebral discs. (See attached Table) In a later chapter, we describe our antibody test results for EBV reactivation in 110 AA patients. All showed some laboratory evidence of past EBV reactivations, and about 70% showed current reactivation.

Our conclusion is that inflammation may simultaneously occur in multiple spinal tissues and be worthy of the label "spinal inflammatory disease." Painful spinal inflammatory conditions may be a component of muti-site, migratory pain disease. EBV R&A may be a causative factor in both multi-site, migratory pain disease and spinal inflammatory diseases.

TABLE

Some Common Labels and MRI Findings in Back Pain Patients with Elevated EBV Antibodies	
Condition Label	MRI Findings
Degenerative disc disease	Discs have shrunk and protrude
Adhesive arachnoiditis	Clumping of nerve roots
Tarlov cysts	Cystic structures in lumbar-sacral canal
Vertebral arthritis	Erosion of vertebrae
Spinal stenosis	Canal narrowed
All the above conditions are caused by chronic inflammation and may simultaneously exist. Spinal inflammation is often caused by EBV reactivation and autoimmunity.	

TABLE

Spinal Conditions Accompanying AA N = 36		
CONDITION	No.	%
Herniated discs	29	80.5
Tarlov cyst	18	50.0
Scoliosis	17	47.2
Spinal fluid leak	15	41.7
Tethered cord	12	33.3
Chiari malformation	5	13.9

Persons in the study reported that these conditions occurred either before or simultaneously with adhesive arachnoiditis. All participants had more than a single condition.

12. EBV Reactivation in Adhesive Arachnoiditis

Lumbar-sacral AA is notoriously known as a disease of IP.[2,4,9] Without vigorous treatment, it is a severe crippling disease. AA occurs when cauda equina nerves become inflamed and glued to the arachnoid lining (inner layer of the spinal canal cover) by adhesions. When this occurs, cauda equina nerves become entrapped in an inflamed, adhesive mass inside the spinal canal. This tragic event not only causes the severest of pain but neurologic impairments of bladder, intestine, sex organs, and lower extremities. If untreated and uncontrolled AA results in paralysis, a bed-bound state, and premature death. Suicide is common.

The great majority of persons who develop AA have one of these predisposing causes or risk factors: (1) heritable connective tissue disorder (e.g. Ehlers-Danlos Syndrome), (2) severe spine, skeletal or head trauma including stroke, (3) autoimmune disease, (4) structural spine abnormality (e.g. scoliosis, ankylosing spondylitis), (5) toxin in spinal fluid caused by a spinal canal puncture or trauma or (6) infectious mononucleosis, Lyme, mycoplasma.

Our studies are very clear in that AA is an "end-of-the-line" disease that develops in a patient with one of the above predisposing conditions or risk factors and is preceded by "multi-site, migratory pain disease" and/or "spinal inflammatory disease." For example, patients with AA almost always give a history of multiple pain sites as described in a previous chapter. AA is always preceded or accompanied by one or more spinal inflammatory conditions that may include herniated discs, Tarlov cysts, tethered cord or spinal fluid leaks. A summary of 36 MRI-documented AA cases with their accompanying spine abnormalities is in the prior chapter. Spinal procedures such as surgery, spinal taps, and epidural injections done for bonafide medical indications may accelerate the development of AA. Simply put, AA is the end of a long unfortunate pathologic pathway (see schemata).

Until now it has never been clear why inflammation and adhesions simultaneously develop in the arachnoid membrane and cauda equina nerves which is necessary to precipitate AA. To determine if EBV may be a causative factor in AA, we reviewed 110 persons with magnetic resonance imaging (MRI) documentation of AA, and who had EBV antibody testing.

In January 2023 we asked persons with documented AA in our study group to take EBV blood tests under supervision of their personal physicians. Testing was done by their local laboratory resource. One-hundred-ten persons submitted their results along with some basic demographic data. There were 94 (85.5%) females and 16 (14.5%) males. Ages ranged from 26 to 80. Table One shows the test results. All were tested for VCA IgG and EBNA IgG antibodies. Ninety-Four (94.3%) showed antibody levels of both antibodies to be above normal range for their testing laboratory. Perhaps significant is that over 50% of the cases of VCA IgG and EBNA IgG had antibody levels above their laboratory's maximal testing threshold suggesting that EBV reactivation had repeatedly taken place in the past. Forty-one patients were tested for early EBNA IgG antibody which is a marker for current EBV reactivation, and 29 (70.7%) were found to be positive.

The 110 study subjects all had one of the predisposing conditions or risk factors for AA such as a heritable connective tissue disease, spine abnormality, or autoimmune disease. All of them also gave a history compatible with multi-site, migratory pain and spinal inflammatory diseases that preceded their development of AA. All suffered SCP or IP and required daily pain relief medications. About 20% said they had experienced infectious mononucleosis. My conclusion is that EBV R&A acted as a catalyst or causative factor in essentially all these patients.

Epstein-Barr Virus (EBV) Antibodies in 110 Patients With Adhesive Arachnoiditis				
		No. Tested	No. + Positive	%
1	EBV Viral Capsid IgG Antibody (VCA)	106	105	99.1
2	EBV Nuclear Antigen IgG Antibody (EBNA)	105	99	94.3
3	EBV Viral Capsid IgM Antibody (VCA IgM)	94	5	5.3
4	Early Nuclear Antigen IgG Antibody (EA-EBNA IgG)	41	29	70.7

A positive test was an antibody level above the laboratory's normal test range. Elevated VCA and EBNA antibodies indicate past reactivation and are considered markers for autoimmunity. EBNA is believed to be the major carrier of EBV autoantibodies. VCA IgM indicates symptomatic active, current infection such as infectious mononucleosis. I am uncertain why five patients tested positive for EBV IgM antibodies other than they may have an unknown active EBV infection. Early-EBNA indicates current reactivation of EBV.

PATHOLOGIC PATHWAY TO ADHESIVE ARACHNOIDITIS

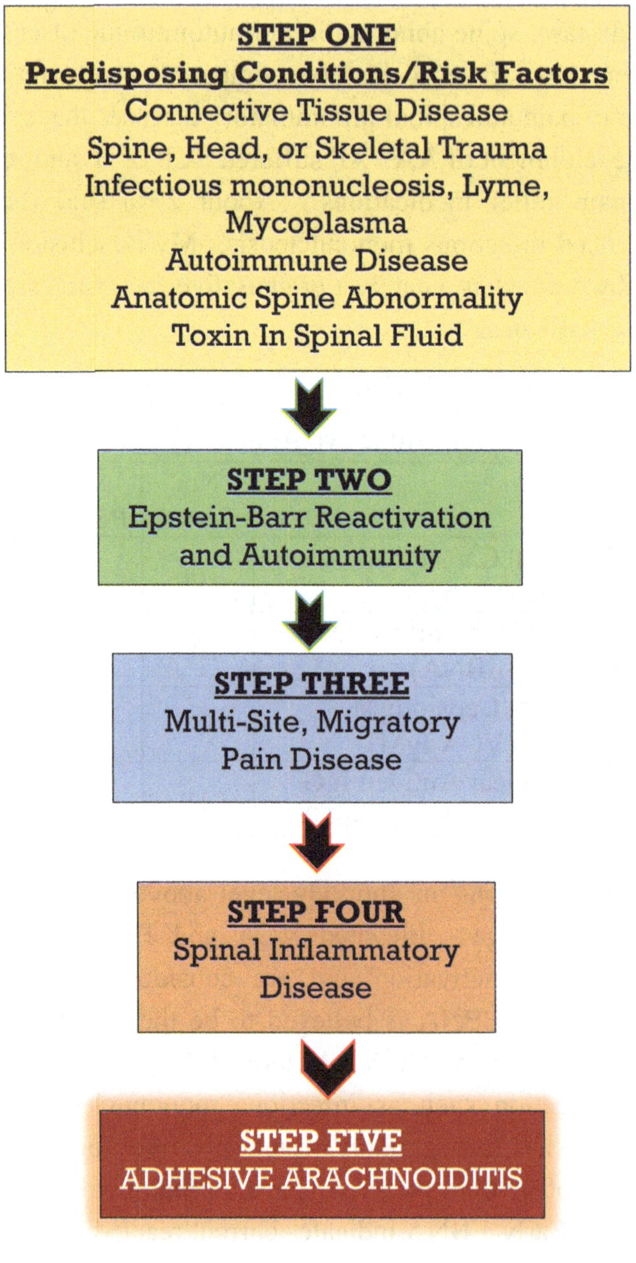

13. How to Determine EBV Reactivation and Autoimmunity

It is relatively simple to determine if EBV R&A is present. The key is to know that EBV R&A may be silent and asymptomatic for a long period before EBV R&A causes a painful disease. Three EBV antibody tests are required to make a diagnosis of EBV R&A.

Unless a blood test is taken a person with diabetes may not know they have the disease until they develop a foot ulcer, stroke, or heart attack. A person with EBV R&A will not know they have a dangerous, asymptomatic disease until they suddenly develop a cancer or painful condition.

Correlation With Clinical Conditions: EBV R&A seems to have a predilection for delicate, thin, tissues like small nerve fibers, fascia, membranes, and intervertebral discs. In our studies the following painful conditions were the first painful conditions experienced by persons who developed multi-site migratory pain and later AA. All had elevated EBV antibodies:

FIRST PAINFUL CONDITION REPORTED IN 110 PATIENTS WITH AA AND EBV R&A

Arthritis	Sciatica
Small fiber neuropathy	Irritable bowel
Migraine	Herniated discs (neck and lumbar)
Carpal tunnel	Temporal mandibular joint (TMJ)
Burning mouth	Loss of teeth
Fibromyalgia	Spinal fluid leaks
Tarlov cysts	Tendonitis
Bursitis	

To make a diagnosis of EBV R&A, it is recommended that a person have two or more of the conditions listed in the attached Table plus quantitative or numerical levels of both VCA IgG and EBNA IgG antibodies at least two times the laboratory upper limit of normal.

Antibody Development and Testing: When EBV first enters the body as well as when it reactivates, it forms these two antibodies are formed to ward off the virus.

#1. Antibody: Targets the capsule of the virus. It is called viral capsid antibody (abbreviated VCA).

#2. Antibody: Targets the nucleus of the virus. It is called "Epstein-Barr nuclear antibody" (abbreviated EBNA).

EXAMPLE OF REACTIVATION Tests are IgG and in units per milliliter	
VCA - NORMAL	PERSON TESTED
0 - 21	420
EBNA - NORMAL	PERSON TESTED
0 - 21	350

All major laboratories now have numerical or quantitative tests given in units per millimeter for these two EBV IgG antibodies. They report numerical levels as normal or elevated just as with a cholesterol or glucose test.

Interpretation: If these two antibodies are significantly elevated above normal, it means that EBV has reactivated one or more times in the past. Significant is defined here as two or more times the normal, upper level for the testing laboratory.

Presumption of Autoimmunity: Reactivation causes EBV to produce autoantibodies, so it is presumed that a high antibody level that is two or more times normal, especially EBNA, is a marker or tracer of autoimmunity.

Current Reactivation: The blood test to determine if a person has current EBV reactivation is called Early Epstein-Barr Nuclear Antibody (IgG) (abbreviated early EBNA). This is important because it calls for consideration of anti-viral, corticosteroid, and other potent viral suppression measures.

It is to be noted that some laboratories now offer an early IgM early nuclear antibody. If positive it indicates that reactivation has started within days or a few weeks prior to the test. This test has little relevance to chronic pain evaluation, however, because it only remains in the serum for a short time period.

Lack of Specific Autoantibody: Currently there is no specific commercial laboratory test for an EBV autoantibody as there is, for example, in rheumatoid arthritis called the RA factor. This, however, may change in the future.

Ancillary Tests: EBV reactivation may sometimes be accompanied by an elevated white blood cell count and/or lymphocyte count. Inflammatory markers such as the erythrocyte sedimentation rate (ESR) or C-reactive protein (CRP) may or may not be elevated. Some interleukins, especially six and ten, may be elevated. The autoimmune nuclear autoantibody (ANA) test may sometimes be positive.

Special EBV Tests: There are some EBV tests for specific non-pain purposes. For example, the IgM VCA antibody is for acute infectious mononucleosis. The polymer chain reaction (PCR) and DNA blood tests are to determine if EBV is in the blood which may occur when severe, acute symptomatic EBV is found in post-transplant cases.

Common Mistakes: A common mistake in EBV testing is to use screening or qualitative (i.e., positive or negative) tests. To determine if EBV R&A is present, numerical or quantitative testing is required. A second mistake is to order the most common test, which is an IgM antibody for acute infectious mononucleosis (VCA IgM). Patients may be erroneously told they don't have EBV, or a "problem" based on this test.

Criteria for Diagnosis: I recommend that a diagnosis of EBV R&A be made when VCA and EBNA IgG antibody levels are at least two times the upper normal, quantitative level of the testing laboratory and that at least two painful medical conditions known to be associated with autoimmunity are present. (See Table) Current reactivation is determined by the early EBNA IgG antibody. It is essential to know if current reactivation is present since it calls for consideration of anti-viral and corticosteroid treatments.

TABLE

The Three EBV IgG Antibody Tests Essential For Determination of Reactivation and Autoimmunity			
	Name of Test	Initials and Antibody	Interpretation of Elevation
1	Epstein-Barr Viral Capsid Antigen Antibody	VCA IgG	There has been one or more past reactivations.
2	Epstein-Barr Nuclear Antigen Antibody	EBNA IgG	Autoantibodies for tissue degeneration, inflammation, and pain are present.
3	Epstein-Barr Early Antigen Nuclear Antibody	EA EBNA IgG	EBV is currently reactivated and causing active autoimmunity.

NOTE: Major laboratories now provide normal ranges for the three EBV IgG antibody tests listed in the Table. I recommend that levels of IgG VCA and EBNA be two or more times the upper normal laboratory level plus pain in two or more anatomic sites to warrant a presumptive diagnosis of EBV R&A.

14. Who Should Be Tested for Reactivation

Unfortunately, EBV R&A can be asymptomatic for a long period before a cancer or painful condition develops. Based on my studies and research, I recommend that some persons with pain conditions be tested for EBV R&A as soon as possible. The sooner that EBV R&A can be determined to be present, the sooner measures can be taken to prevent the worst of consequences. Here are my recommendations for four groups of pain patients who should be tested for EBV R&A.

1. Any person who has had constant pain for over 90 days and must take medication each day to relieve pain.

2. Any person who has "multi-site, migratory pain disease" or "spinal inflammatory disease."

3. Any person with chronic pain who has had infectious mononucleosis, Lyme, or mycoplasma infection.

4. Any person who has a connective tissue disease (e.g., Ehlers-Danlos or Marfan syndrome) and develops a painful anatomic site.

There is the erroneous belief among some patients and medical practitioners that symptomatic pain relief measures will treat the underlying causes of pain including EBV R&A. Even if symptomatic pain relief is excellent with opioids, electrical stimulator, or surgery, the EBV pathologic, autoimmune process is still active, persistent, and may later progress to a cancer or likely continue to deteriorate the painful condition.

Although it may not be possible to totally extinguish EBV since it is a natural parasite from the human body or remove all autoantibodies, EBV R&A can almost always be contained and controlled so that cancer or painful diseases won't either develop, progress, or shorten a person's life.

15. Treatment of EBV Reactivation

Treatment measures for EBV R&A fall into three categories: (1) inhibition of reactivation, (2) suppression of inflammation, and (3) reduction of viral load.

Inhibition of Reactivation

Some innovative researchers have tested a large number of medicinals in laboratory settings to determine which ones inhibit EBV reactivation. A Table of these agents with references to their testing source is in this chapter. Inhibiting reactivation is an essential first step in the control and containment of EBV R&A. If reactivation is stopped, tissue infiltration, toxic emissions, and possibly the autoimmune process may eventually reduce or cease because additional or replacement viruses will not be available. It is my recommendation that a person who meets the criteria (elevated antibodies plus two painful conditions) take two or more medicinals to inhibit reactivation.

Suppression of Inflammation and Tissue Destruction

The painful conditions caused by EBV R&A are initiated by inflammation in tissues including the glial cells in the CNS. EBV R&A seems to predominantly affect nerve tissue in and outside the CNS.[44,48,67] At this time, I recommend intermittent, low dosage use of a corticosteroid and the potent CNS anti-inflammatory, ketorolac. A simple and safe regimen is prednisone (5mg), methylprednisolone (4mg) or dexamethasone (0.5 to .75 mg) given one to three times a week. Ketorolac can be taken orally or by injection. A starting safe regimen is 10 to 30 mg every 1 to 2 weeks. Anti-inflammatory agents such as celecoxib or diclofenac may be efficacious for painful conditions whose anatomic location is outside the spine. Outside of ketorolac, inflammatory agents are inconsistent in crossing the blood brain barrier and achieving adequate spinal fluid levels.

Suppression of glial cell induced neuroinflammation must be a component of treatment to eliminate such central symptoms as hyperalgesia, pain sensitization, and cognitive impairments.[48] Methylprednisolone and dexamethasone but not prednisone have been shown to suppress glial cell activation and neuroinflammation.[62,96] Minocycline, metformin, and pentoxifylline will suppress glial cell neuroinflammation.

I consider it essential to attempt a counterbalance to the tissue destruction of EBV R&A. A failure to do this simply means that autoantibodies can continually destroy tissues and increase pain, unabated. I recommend protein be eaten daily (many persons in modern society rarely eat fish, poultry, beef, lamb, or eggs) and a regular collagen supplement. Also, I highly recommend polypeptides and anabolic hormones. Thymosin is both a hormonal substance and peptide that is recommended. Colostrum and deer antler lining ("velvet") are multi-hormone supplements that have anabolic properties. The natural neurosteroids, DHEA and nandrolone, and the anabolic hormones, human chorionic gonadotropin (HCG) and human growth hormone (HGH), should be considered in a patient who is losing muscle mass, developing paralysis, or has incessant spinal fluid leaks.[24,58,81]

Reduction of Viral Load

Three medicinals have emerged as popular agents for viral load reduction. They have different mechanisms of action. One is low dose naltrexone whose mechanism is primarily to enhance natural immune functions. The second is a medicinal called Monolaurin™ which is a derivative of coconut oil. Its mechanism is unclear, but some observers believe it is virucidal. The third is one of these three anti-viral agents: acyclovir (Zovirax®), valacyclovir (Valtrex®), and famciclovir (Famvir®). The dosage of acyclovir is 400 to 1000 mg a day and valacyclovir and famciclovir is 500 to 1000 mg a day. If antivirals are attempted, a trial of 30 days is usually sufficient to determine if they are effective. Some physicians are attempting combinations of antiviral agents and low dose, long-term therapy. Anti-parasitic agents may also be useful.

Combination Therapy

Studies to date with antiviral agents have almost all been directed at fibromyalgia with the belief that the offending viruses are herpes I and II and not EBV. Antiviral agents used alone haven't been consistently successful. However, one well done and underappreciated study has shown that a combination of famciclovir (Famvir®) and celecoxib to be safe and efficacious in the treatment of fibromyalgia. This study was headed by William Pridgen and is remarkable in that it studied 143 fibromyalgia patients at twelve different clinical sites. The authors believed they were targeting Herpes I and II and recognized that there are overlapping painful conditions associated with fibromyalgia. The most important aspect of this study coincides with my experience in that a combination of agents that have different targets of treatment bring the best results.

Due to the urgency to suppress EBV R&A, a number of investigators are searching for new agents. Recently spironolactone has been publicized as an agent that may reduce viral load. At the time this book is being written, there are no clinical reports on its effectiveness, but, hopefully, this inexpensive and safe drug will prove effective.

Current Reactivation

The early Epstein-Barr nuclear antigen antibody (Early EBNA) is the most essential test because it is the test for the presence of current reactivation. Simply put, if the early EBNA IgG antibody is elevated above normal, it means that the person has an active virus that is likely infiltrating tissue, creating toxins, and fostering autoimmunity.[10,55,103] Efforts must be made to revert current reactivation to inactive. Persons who have elevated early EBNA antibodies should be considered for anti-viral agents and corticosteroids in addition to agents that inhibit reactivation. It is advised that regular, periodic early EBNA IgG tests be taken to determine if treatment measures to cease reactivation are successful.

The early EBNA IgG antibody R&A will show a reduction in blood level if the treatment is finding its mark and reactivation is shutting down. Interestingly, VCA and EBNA IgG antibodies may not show any reduction in blood level with treatment, because they are protective antibodies that may likely remain elevated for life.

Treatments for EBV R&A are not substitutes or alternatives for treatments used for any disease, condition, or symptom. The measures here are conjunctive or in addition to standard therapies such as analgesics, peptides, or hormones. In the author's experience, treatment of EBV R&A will usually reduce the dosage and frequency of symptomatic pain medications but will not usually obviate a total need for them.

In summary, EBV R&A treatments should include measures directed at inhibiting reactivation, suppressing tissue inflammation, and reducing viral load. The most critical EBV test in patients with EBV R&A is early EBNA IgG antibody since this test represents current reactivation and a need for aggressive attempts to halt reactivation.

TABLE

MEDICINALS FOR INHIBITION OF EPSTEIN-BARR VIRUS REACTIVATION

Vitamin C
Vitamin D
Resveratrol
Luteolin
Astragalus
Curcumin
Andrographis
Cimetidine
Selenium
Zinc
Lysine

The medicinals listed here have been shown in laboratory testing to have inhibitory activity on EBV reactivation.

References

1. Andre G, Trompet E, Snoeck R. Novel therapeutics for Epstein-Barr virus. *Molecules* 2019;24:997-1009.
2. Eladwy RA, Vu HT, Shah R, et al. The fight against the carcinogenic Epstein-Barr virus: gut microbiota, natural medicines and beyond. *Int J Mol Sci* 2023;24:1716-1725.
3. Kerr J. Epstein-Barr virus (EBV) reactivation and therapeutic inhibitors. *J Clin Pathol* 2019;0:1-8.

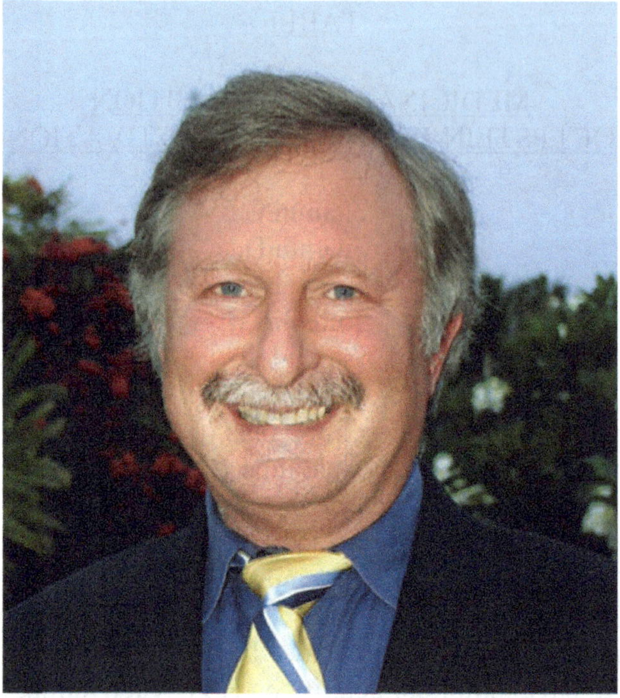

Dr. Jacob Teitelbaum has been the leading physician in this century to develop comprehensive treatment protocols for persons who have multi-site, migratory pain disease. His methods incorporate a combination of nutrition, herbal, hormonal, and anti-viral measures.

Summary

EBV R&A should rightfully be labelled a disease. It attacks tissues in a random and unpredictable manner causing degeneration, inflammation, and pain. EBV now causes at least 2% of the world's cancers. Given its ability to produce pain in every tissue of the body, an appropriate name for this complication is "multi-site, migratory pain disease." EBV R&A has a predilection for fine delicate tissues such as small nerve fibers, fascia, and membranes. It has an affinity for the brain and spinal cord and may simultaneously produce inflammation in glial cells, intervertebral discs, cauda equina, and arachnoid membrane. This development should rightfully be called "spinal inflammatory disease." EBV R&A appeared to be a causative factor or catalyst in the development of adhesive arachnoiditis.

Based on cumulated information to date, it seems clear that every person with severe chronic or intractable pain should be evaluated and tested for EBV R&A. If present, the patient should embark upon specific preventive and treatment measures. In almost all cases, EBV R&A can be effectively controlled and contained. Testing and treatment of EBV R&A is easily done and will enhance the ongoing treatment of almost every pain patient.

Glossary

Adhesive Arachnoiditis: An intraspinal canal inflammatory disorder in which a clump or mass of cauda equina nerves are glued by adhesions to the arachnoid-dural covering of the spinal canal.

Antibody: A substance produced by B lymphocytes in response to an offending antigen. There are five antibody classes known as immunoglobulins: IgA, IgD, IgE, IgG, and IgM. IgM is the earliest antibody produced against a virus but disappears from the serum after a short time period. IgG is the antibody produced by the body for long-term protection.

Arachnoiditis-non-adhesive: Inflammation of the arachnoid layer of the spinal canal covering (meninges) without any nerves adhered to it. This condition cannot specifically be identified by MRI. It is a clinical diagnosis based on signs, symptoms, and laboratory tests.

Autoinfection: Disease condition including pain and polymyositis that stem from an internal parasite usually found in the intestine.

Autoimmune Disease: A disease in which a person's own tissues are mistaken by an autoantibody or other element to be an outside invader such as a virus or bacteria and attacks and destroys one's own tissues.

Autoantibody: A globulin protein that attacks normal tissues to cause inflammation, tissue destruction, scarring, pain, and cancer.

Autoimmunity: An internal disease process that attacks and destroys tissue by an autoantibody.

Bioelectricity: The electricity formed in tissue that fosters metabolism, muscular movement, and neurologic functions.

Cauda equina: About two dozen nerves that emanate from the spinal cord at the level of thoracic 12(T-12) or lumbar 1 (L-1) vertebrae and are suspended in spinal fluid. The term nerve roots is often applied rather than nerves.

Chronic Pain: A pain that persists longer than the usual healing time of about ninety days.

Collagen: A strong fibrous insoluble protein found in connective tissue including the dermis, tendons, ligaments, fascia, bone, cartilage, nerves, and membranes.

Connective Tissue Disorder: A genetic disease in which collagen in tissues is deficient and weakens the tissues which may result in inflammation, adhesions, scarring, and pain.

Corticoid or Corticosteroid: A pharmaceutical that is chemically related to cortisone.

Dormant: State in which a parasitic virus is in tissues but inactive and not causing any pathologic complications.

Ehlers-Danlos Syndrome (EDS): A genetic connective tissue disorder named after two physicians who first described the condition. The most common form is hypermobile.

Epstein-Barr Autoimmunity: An internal disease state in which EBV has reactivated and produced autoantibodies or equivalent process that causes tissue inflammation, destruction, pain, and cancer.

Epstein Barr Virus: A virus of the herpes class (No. 4) that is normally an innocuous human parasite but may reactivate and produce an autoimmune disorder and a number of pathologic conditions including some cancers and painful diseases. Named after the scientists who discovered the virus in a cancer known as Burkitt's lymphoma.

Failed Back Surgery Syndrome: Condition assigned to persons who had spine surgery that failed to relieve the pain for which surgery was done.

Fibromyalgia: Diffuse pain in muscle groups and their fibrous connections to ligaments, fascia, and bone.

Herb: A medicinal that comes from a plant or botanical.

Hypermobile: The ability to over-extend skin, joints, and extremities beyond normal range.

Hypermobile Spectrum Disorder: A group of about a dozen, rare genetic collagen deficient, connective tissue conditions that are related to but don't qualify as hypermobile Ehlers-Danlos Syndrome.

Inflammation: Tissue that is red, hot, degenerating tissue followed by pain and functional impairment.

Immunoglobulin-IgG: A protein antibody that is made by B lymphocytes and plasma cells that help the body fight infection.

Immunoglobulin-M: First antibody to appear when the body is exposed to an antigen. It disappears after a short time period.

Intractable Pain: Constant, incurable pain that may produce cardiovascular, respiratory, endocrine, and metabolic complications.

In Vivo: Growth of tissue or a microbe in the body.

In Vitro: Growth of tissue or a microbe outside the body as in a test tube, plate, or dish.

Latent Phase: A state after initial infection when a virus is quiet, silent, and harmless. Same meaning as dormant.

Lumbar Spine: A lower back section of the spine consisting of five lumbar vertebrae levels being designated L1 through L5 with L1 being the topmost vertebrae.

Lymphocyte: A white blood cell which makes up about 25% of the body's total white blood cells. There are two main types: The B cell makes antibodies for immune protection and T cells that help B lymphocytes and/or remove cells that contain an offending infectious agent.

Lymphoma: A cancer of lymph tissues which may cause enlargement of lymph nodes.

Lytic Phase: Period in which a virus is multiplying or replicating by dividing itself.

Marfan Syndrome: A hereditary disorder of connective tissue, bones, muscles, ligaments, and skeletal structures. It is characterized by a tall lean body with long fingers, toes, joint flexibility, and flat feet.

Meninges: This is the covering of the brain and spinal canal consisting of three layers: dura, arachnoid, and pia mater. In the lumbar-sacral region of the spine, the spinal canal covering primarily consists of an inside layer, the arachnoid, and an outer layer, dura. The word "covering" is preferentially used in this book rather than meninges or theca to simplify understanding.

Multi-Site, Migratory Pain Disease: Condition in which pain simultaneously occurs in multiple anatomic sites and the pains, overtime, will migrate to additional or different anatomical sites.

Natural: A medicinal that is made in the human body.

Polymyositis: Inflammation and pain of many muscles often called myofascial syndrome.

Precursor: An antecedent medical condition that leads to another or a chemical substance that makes another by metabolism.

Reactivation: A change from a dormant, carrier state to one in which the virus begins to duplicate and becomes an active infectious agent that can produce painful diseases and cancer.

Receptor: A molecular tissue site composed of protein which receives a neurotransmitter or biochemical and then creates some function.

Sarcoma: Generic name for a cancer that arises in bone, muscle, or other connective tissues.

Spinal canal: The spinal canal is a structure like a closed pipe that carries the spinal fluid. The fluid is primarily produced in the brain and flows down the canal on one side and flows back up to the brain to be diverted into lymph nodes and the general blood and lymphatic systems. The word canal is preferentially used here to simplify understanding.

Spinal Inflammatory Disease: Inflammation that simultaneously occurs in multiple spinal tissues which may include vertebrae, intervertebral discs, ligamentum flavum, cauda equina nerves, filum terminale, arachnoid membrane, and the dural layer of the spinal canal cover.

Spinal Tap: A puncture of the spinal canal to either place a substance inside the canal or withdraw fluid.

Spine: Refers to the entire spine including vertebrae, intervertebral discs, spinal canal, cord inside the canal, and cauda equina nerves.

Vector: A person, animal, or insect such as a mosquito that carries and transmits a disease.

Selected Bibliography

1. Bartemus, J. The Autoimmune Answer. Best Seller Publishing, Pasadena, CA, 2020.

2. Burkitt DP, Wright DH. Burkitt's Lymphoma. E & S Livingstone, Edinburgh & London, 1970.

3. Eliaz I. The Survival Paradox: Reversing the Hidden Cause of Aging and Chronic Disease Lioncrest, 2022.

4. Eran E. Epstein-Barr Virus Treatment Handbook. Coppell, Texas, 2024.

5. Hoagland RJ. Infectious Mononucleosis. Grune & Stratton, New York & London, 1967.

6. Jefferies, WM. Safe Uses of Cortisol. Charles C. Thomas Ltd, Springfield, Ill, 3rd ed, 2004.

7. Kines K. The Epstein-Barr virus solution. Coppell, TX, 2023.

8. Lam M, Lam D. Adrenal Fatigue Syndrome. Adrenal Institute Press, Loma Linda, CA, 2012.

9. Nakazawa, DJ. The Autoimmune Epidemic. Simon & Schuster, New York, 2008.

10. Rawls B. The cellular wellness solution. First Do No Harm Pub, Raleigh, NC, 2022.

11. Robertson ES. Epstein-Barr Virus. Calister Academic Press, Norfolk, England, 2005.

12. Talbott, S. The Cortisol Connection. Hunter House, Berkeley, CA, 2002.

13. Teitelbaum J. The Fatigue and Fibromyalgia Solution. Avery, New York, 2013.

14. Teitelbaum J. Pain Free 1-2-3. McGraw-Hill, New York, 2005.

15. Teitelbaum J. From Fatigue to Fantastic. Avery, New York, 2020, 4th ed.

16. Vasquez, A. Pain Revolution for Migraine and Fibromyalgia. International College of Human Nutrition and Functional Medicine, Charleston, SC, 2016.

17. William A. Medical Medium: Secrets Behind Chronic and Mystery Illness and How to Finally Heal. Hay House Inc. Carlsbad, Calif., USA, 2021.

18. Wilson, JL. Adrenal Fatigue: The 21st Century Stress Syndrome. Smart Publications, Petaluma, CA 2002.

References

1. Aalto SM, Linnavuori K, Peltola, et al. Immunocostivation of Epstein-Barr virus due to cytomegalovirus disease. *J Med Virol* 1998;56:186-91.
2. Aldrete JA. Suspecting and diagnosing arachnoiditis. *Pract Pain Mgt* 2006;16:74-87.
3. Alspaugh MA, Henle G, Lennette E, et al. Elevated levels of antibodies to Epstein-Barr virus antigens in sera and synovial fluids of patients with rheumatoid arthritis. *J Clin Invest* 1981;67:1134-1140.
4. Anderson TL, Morris JM, Wald JT, et al. Imaging appearance of advanced chronic adhesive arachnoiditis: A retrospective review. *Am J Roentgenol* 2017;209:648-655.
5. Andre G, Trompet E, Snoeck R. Novel therapeutics for Epstein-Barr virus. *Molecules* 2019;24:997-1009.
6. Apkarian AV, Sosa Y, Sont S, et al. Chronic back pain is associated with decreased prefrontal and thalamic gray matter density. *J Neurosci* 2004;24:10410-10415.
7. Baken JS. Epstein-Barr-Virus induced glomerulonephritis. *Tidsske Nor Laegeforen* 1980;100:558-560.
8. Bashir K, Lipton RB, Achina S, et al. Migraine and structural changes in the brain. *Neurology* 2013;81:1-9.
9. Bilello J, Tennant F. Patterns of chronic inflammation in extensively treated patients with arachnoiditis and chronic intractable pain. *Postgrad Med* 2016;92:1-5.
10. Binne UK, Amun W, Furrell PJ. Promotor sequence required for reactivation of Epstein-Barr virus from latency. *J Virology* 2002;76:10282-10289.
11. Birkenfeld P, Haratz N, Klein G, et al. Cross reactivity between the BNA-LP107 peptide, collagen, and keratin: implications for the pathogenesis of rheumatoid arthritis. *Clin Immunol & Immunopath* 1990;54:14-25.

12. Bjornevik K, Cortese M, Healy BC, et al, et al. Longitudinal analysis reveals high prevalence of Epstein-Barr virus associated with multiple sclerosis. *Science* 2022;375:296-301.
13. Bonor RA, Weinstein D, Sommer JR, et al. Virus of avian myeloblastosis XVII morphology of progressive virus myeloblast interactions in vitro. *US Nat Cancer Inst Monog* 1960;4:251-290.
14. Bronz G, Benedetto P, Zanetti SM, et al. Bilateral upper eyelid swelling (Hoagland sign) in Epstein-Barr infectious mononucleosis: prospective experience. *Infection* 2023;51:471-474.
15. Brunell PA, Gershon AA, Uduman SA, et al. Varicella-zoster immunoglobulins during varicella, latency, and zoster. *J Infect Dis* 1975;132:49-54.
16. Buchwald D, Garrity D. Chronic fatigue, fibromyalgia and chemical sensitivity: overlapping disorders. *Arch Intern Med 1994;154:2049-2053.*
17. Buckalew N, Haut MW, Morrow L, et al. Chronic pain is associated with brain volume loss in older adults: preliminary evidence. *Pain Med* 2008;9:240-248.
18. Burkitt DP. Primary hydrocele and its treatment: a review of 200 cases. *Lancet* 1951;1:1341-1343.
19. Burkitt DP. A sarcoma involving the jaws of African children. *Brit J Surg* 1958;46:218-223.
20. Burkitt DP, O'Connor GT. Malignant lymphoma in African children: a clinical syndrome. *Cancer* 1961;14:258-269.
21. Campana WM. Schwann cells: activated peripheral glia and their role in neuropathic pain. *Brain Behav Immun* 2007;21:522-527.
22. Catalano MA, Carson DA, Sloven SF, et al. Antibodies to Epstein-Barr virus-determined antigens in normal subjects and in patients with seropositive rheumatoid arthritis. *Proc Nat Acad Sci* 1979;76:5825-5828.
23. Cauda F, Palerno S, Costa T, et al. Gray matter alterations in chronic pain: a network-oriented meta-analytic approach. *Neuroimage Clin* 2014;16:676-685.

24. Chang DM, Chu SJ, Chen HC, et al. Dehydroepiandrosterone suppresses interleukin 10 synthesis in women with systemic lupus erythematosus. *Ann Rheum Dis* 2004;63:1623-1620.
25. Clark EH, Ashley P, Shandera WX. Epstein-Barr virus & infectious mononucleosis in *Current Medical Diagnosis and Treatment*. Ed Papdakis MA, McPhee JJ, Rabow MW. McQuaid KP. *McGraw Hill*, New York 20241,371-1373.
26. Cohen JL. Epstein-Barr Virus infection. *New Eng J* Med 2000;343:481-492.
27. Cohen JL, Wang W, Mannick J, et al. Epstein-Barr virus nuclear protein 2 is a key determinant of lymphocyte transformation. *Prac Natl Acad Sci USA* 1989;86:9558-9562.
28. Coskum O, Sener K, Kilic S, et al. Stress-related Epstein-Barr virus reactivation. *Clin Exp Med* 2010;10:15-20.
29. Duan Y, et al. Immune cell infiltration and the genes associated with ligamentum flavum hypertrophy: identification and validation. *Front Cell Dev Biol* 2022;10:91478.
30. Eladwy RA, Vu HT, Shah R, et al. The fight against the carcinogenic Epstein-Barr virus: gut microbiota, natural medicines and beyond. *Int J Mol Sci* 2023;24:1716-1725.
31. Epstein MA, Barr YM, Achang BC. Virus particles in cultured lymphocytes from Burkitt's lymphoma. *Lancet 1964;1:702-703.*
32. Fine PG. Long-term consequences of chronic pain: mounting evidence for pain as a neurologic disease and parallels with other chronic disease states. *Pain* Med 2011;12:996-1004.
33. Fischer GA. Studies of the culture of leukemic cells in vitro. *Annals NY Acad Sci* 1958;76:673-680.
34. Gome K, Goldman RD. Corticosteroids for infectious mononucleosis. *Can FAM Physician* 2023;2:101-102.
35. Gordon MP. Corticosteroid treatment of infectious mononucleosis in a military population. *Military Medicine* 1968;133:303-305.

36. Gould GM, Pyle WL. Autoinfection in Cyclopedia of Practical Medicine and Surgery. *P Blakiston's Son & Co.*, Philadelphia, 1900.
37. Harley JB, Chan X, Pujato M, et a. Transaction factors operate across disease loci, with EBNA2 implicated in autoimmunity. *Nat Genet* 2018;50:699-707.
38. Harrow T. Epstein-Barr virus could be a cause of multiple autoimmune disorders. *VA Research Currents* April 18, 2018.
39. Henle G, Henle N, Diehl V. Relation of Burkitt's tumor associated herpes type virus to infectious mononucleosis. *Proc Natl Acad* Sci 1968;59:94-101.
40. Henle G, Henle W. Immunofluorescence in cells derived from Burkitt's lymphomas. *J Bact* 1966;91:1248-1256.
41. Henle G, Henle W, Klein G, et al. Antibodies to early Epstein-Barr virus-induced antigens in Burkitt's lymphoma. *J Nat Cancer Inst* 1971;46:861-871.
42. Henle W, Henle G. Epstein-Barr virus-related serology in Hodgkin's disease. *Nat Cancer Inst Monograph* 1973;36:79-84.
43. Henle G, Henle W, Diehl V. Relation of Burkitt's tumor associated herpes type virus to infectious mononucleosis. *Proc Natl Acad Sci* 1968;59:94-101.
44. Hirshout Y, Glade P, Viera LO, et al. Sarcoidosis, another disease associated with serologic evidence for herpes-like infection. *New Eng J Med* 1970;283:502-506.
45. Hoagland RJ. Infectious mononucleosis. *Amer J Med* 1952;13:158-171.
46. Hoagland RJ, Henson HM. Splenic rupture in infectious mononucleosis. *Ann Intern Med* 1957;46:1184.
47. Houen G, Trier NH. Epstein-Barr virus and systemic autoimmune disease. *Front Immunol* 2020;11:1-13.
48. Hsu D, Malefytro W, Fiorentino DF, et al. Expression of interleukin-10 activity by Epstein-Barr virus protein BCRF 1. *Science* 1990;250:830-832.
49. Hung AL, Lim M, Doshi TC. Targeting cytokines for treatment of neuropathic pain. *Scand J Pain* 2017;17:287-293.

50. Indari O, Tiwari D, Tanwar M, et al. Early biomolecular changes in brain microvascular endothelial cells under Epstein-Barr virus influence: A Raman microspectroscopic investigation. *Integr Biol* 2022;14:89-97.
51. Indari O, Jakhomola S, Pathak DK, et al. Comparative account of biomolecular changes post Epstein Barr virus infection of the neuronal and glial cells using Raman microspectroscopy. *ACS Chem Neurosci* 2022;13:1627-1637.
52. Jakhmola S, Jha HM. Glial cell response to Epstein Barr Virus infection: a plausible contribution to virus-associated inflammatory reactions in the brain. *Virology* 2021;559:182-195.
53. Jauregui-Huerta F, Ruvalcaba-Delgadillo Y, Gonzales-Casteneda R, et al. Responses of glia cells to stress and glucocorticoids. *Curr Immunol Rev* 2010;6:195-204.
54. Javida E, Magnus T. Autoimmunity after ischemic stroke and brain injury. *Front Immunol* 2019;10:1-12.
55. Jha HC, Pei Y, Robertson ES. Epstein-Barr virus: disease linked to infection and transformation. 2016;7:1-16.
56. Johansson B, Klein G, Henle W, et al. Epstein-Barr virus (EBV) associated antibody patterns in malignant lymphoma and leukemia. I. Hodgkins disease. *Int J Cancer* 1970;6:450-462.
57. Johansson B, Klein G, Henle W, et al. Epstein-Barr virus (EBV) associated antibody patterns in malignant lymphoma and leukemia. II. chronic lymphatic leukemia and lymphocytic lymphoma. *Int J Cancer* 1971;8:475-486.
58. Jones KJ. Gonadal steroids and neuronal regeneration: a therapeutic role. *Adv Neurol* 1993;59:227-240.
59. Katz, BZ. Infectious mononucleosis in *Conn's Current Therapy* 2024, ed. Kellerman RD, Rakel DP, Heidelbaugh JJ, Lee FM. *Elsevier* Philadelphia, 626-627.
60. Kenney SC, Mertz JE. Regulation of the latent-lytic switch in Epstein-Barr virus. *Semin Cancer Biol* 2014;26:60-68.
61. Kerr J. Epstein Barr Virus (EBV) reactivation and therapeutic inhibitors. *J Clin Pathol* 2019;0:1-8.

62. Kiefer R, Kreutzberg GW. Effects of dexamethasone on microglial activation in vitro. *J Neuroimmunology* 1991;34:99-108.
63. Kiguchi N, et al. Chemokines and cytokines in neuroinflammation leading to neuropathic pain. *Curr Opinion Pharmacol* 2012;12:55-61.
64. Li YL, Wang JY, Lil K, et al. Epstein-Barr virus to be a trigger of autoimmune glial fibrillary acidic protein astrocytopathy. *CNS Neurosci Ther* 2023;29:4139-4146.
65. Libert N, Bigailon C, Chargari C, et al. Epstein-Barr virus reactivation in critically ill immunocompetent patients. *Biomed J* 2015;38:70-76.
66. Lofgren S. Concepts of sarcoidosis. *Pasth Med Scand* 1964;425:1-6.
67. Maier A, Kapfenberger R, Katano I, et al. Nonregional small fiber neuropathy in cases of autoimmune autonomic neuropathy. J Neurol 2022;269:6648-6654.
68. Meisel C, Schwab JM, Prass K, et al. Central nervous system injury-induced immune deficiency syndrome. *Nat Rev Neurosci* 2005;6:775-786.
69. Mika J, Zychowska M, Popiolek-Barczy K, et al. Importance of glial activation in neuropathic pain. *Eur J Pharmacol* 2013;716:106-119.
70. Milligan ED, Watkins LR. Pathological and protective roles of glia in chronic pain. Nat Rev Neurosci 2009;10:23- 36.
71. Nagata K, Hayashi K. Epstein-Barr virus reactivation-induced immunoglobulin production: significance on autoimmunity. *Microorganisms* 2020;8:1875-1890.
72. Nahmias AJ, Roizman B. Infection with herpes simplex viruses 1 and 2. *N Engl J Med* 1973;289:667-674.
73. Nakamura M, Burasteros F, Vaki Y, et al. Proving the normal and autoimmune B cell repertoire with Epstein-Barr virus, frequency of B cells producing monoreactive high affinity autoantibodies in patients with Hashimoto's disease and systemic lupus erythematosus. *J Immunnol* 1998;141:4165-4172.

74. Ngou J, Graafland H, Segondy M. Antibodies against polypeptides of purified Epstein-Barr virus in serum from patients with connective tissue diseases. *J Autoimmun* 1992;5:243-249.
75. Niederman JC, McCollum W, Henle G, et al. Infectious mononucleosis: clinical manifestations in relation to Epstein-Barr virus. *J Am Med Assoc* 1968;203:139-143,
76. O'Callaghan JP, Sriram, Miller DB. Defining "neuroinflammation". *Ann NY Acad Sci* 2008;1139:318-330.
77. Ogra PL, Kerr-Grant D, Umana G, et al. Antibody response in serum and nasopharynx after naturally acquired and vaccine-induced infection with rubella virus. *N Eng J Med* 1971;285:1333-1339.
78. Okano M, Kawa K, Kimura H, et al. Proposed guidelines for diagnosing chronic active Epstein-Barr infection. *Am J Hematol* 2005;80:64-69.
79. Pridgen WL, Duffy C, Gendreau JF, et al. A famciclovir and celecoxib combination treatment is safe and efficacious in the treatment of fibromyalgia. *J Pain Res* 2017;10:451-460.
80. Raffaeli W, Arando E. Pain as a disease: an overview. *J Pain* Res 2017;10:2003-2008.
81. Reddy DS. Neurosteroids: endogenous role in the human brain and therapeutic potentials. *Prog Brain Res* 2010;186:13-137.
82. Rhodes G, Pumpold H, Kurki P, et al. Autoantibosies in infectious mononucleosis have specificity for the glycine-alanine repeating region of the Epstein-Barr virus nuclear antigen. *J Exp Med 1987;165:1026-1040.*
83. Rickinson AB. Chronic symptomatic Epstein-Barr virus infection. *Immunol Today* 1986;7:13-14.
84. Rodriguez-Raecke R, Niemeier A, Ihler K, et al. Brain gray matter decrease in chronic pain is the consequence and not the cause of pain. *J Neurosci* 2009;29:13746-13750.

85. Ross CAC, McDaid R. Specific IgM antibody in serum of patients with herpes zoster infections. *Br Med J* 1972;4:522-523.
86. Seminowicz DA, Labus JS, Bueller JA, et al. Regional gray matter density changes in brains of patients with irritable bowel syndrome. *Gastroenterology* 2010;139:48-57.
87. Seminowicz DA, Wideman TH, Naso L, et al. Effective treatment of chronic low back pain in humans reverses abnormal brain anatomy and function. *J Neuroscience* 2011;31:7540-7550.
88. Soni N, Ora R, Sing P, et al. Unpacking the CNS manifestations of Epstein-Barr virus: an imaging perspective. *Amer J Neurorad* 2023;44:1002-1008.
89. Strannegard O, Holm SE, Hermudson S, et al. Case of apparent reinfection with rubella. *Lancet* 1970;1:240-241.
90. Strauss SE. The chronic mononucleosis syndrome. *J Infect Dis* 1988;157:405-412.
91. Sumaya CV, Henle W, Henle G, et al. Seroepidemiologic study of Epstein-Barr virus infections in a rural community. *J Infect Disease* 1975;131:403-408.
92. Sumaya, CV. Endogenous reactivation of Epstein-Barr virus infection. *J Infect Dis* 1977;135:374-379.
93. Sunderson B, Shirafkan F, Ripperger K, et al. The role of viral infections in the onset of autoimmune diseases. *Viruses* 2023;15:782-814.
94. Sutton RN, Emond RT, Thomas DB, et al. The occurrence of autoantibodies in infectious mononucleosis. *Clin Exp Immunol* 1974;17:427-436.
95. Takahashi H, Sugura T, Okazimo Y, et al. Inflammatory cytokines in the herniated disc of the lumbar spine. Spine 1996;21:218-224.
96. Takedo K, Sawamura S, Sekiyama H, et al. Effect of methylprednisolone on neuropathic pain and spinal glial activation in rats. *Anesthesiology* 2004;100:1249-1257.
97. Teitelbaum J. Effective treatment for chronic fatigue syndrome and fibromyalgia: an overview and 35

treatments for tough cases. *Townsend Letter* Nov 2015:56-59.

98. Teitelbaum JE, Bird B, Greenfield RM, et al. Effective treatment of chronic fatigue syndrome and fibromyalgia-randomized, double-blind, placebo-controlled, intent to study. *J of Chron Fatigue Synd* 2000;8:3-15.
99. Tennant F, Hermann L. Intractable or chronic pain: there is a difference. *West J Med* 2000;173:306.
100. Tennant F. The physiologic effects of pain on the endocrine system. *Pain* Ther 2013;2:75-86.
101. Tennant FS. The glomerulonephritis of infectious mononucleosis. *Texas Rpts Biol* Med 1969;26:603-612.
102. Thompson SJ, Pitcher MH, Stone LS, et al. Chronic neuropathic pain reduces opioid receptor availability with associated anhedonia in rat. *Pain* 2018;159:1856-1866.
103. Thurley-Lawson DA, Gross A. Persistence of the Epstein-Barr virus and the urging of associated lymphomas. *N Engl J Med* 2004;350:1328-1337.
104. Tiwari D, Mittal N. Unraveling the links between neurodegeneration and Epstein-Barr virus-mediated cell cycle dysregulation. *Curr Res Neurobiol* 2023;3:2665-2945.
105. Tsai YT, Chiang BL, Kao YF, et al. Detection of Epstein-Barr virus and cytomegalovirus genome in white cells from patients with juvenile rheumatoid arthritis and childhood systemic lupus erythematosus. *Intern Arch Allergy Immunol* 1995;106:235-240.
106. Tsuda M, Beggs S, Salter MW, et al. Microglia and intractable chronic pain. *Glia* 2012;61:55-61.
107. Upchurch KS, Jonathan K. Evolution of treatment for rheumatoid arthritis. *Rheumatology* 2012;51:28-36.
108. Vaughn JH. The Epstein-Barr virus in autoimmunity. *Springer Semin Immunopathol* 1995;17:203-230.
109. Wang L, Wang FS, Gershwin ME. Human autoimmune disease: a comprehensive update. *J Intern Med* 2015;278:369-395.

110. Wahren B, Carlen E, Espmark A, et al. Antibodies to various herpes viruses in sera from patients with sarcoidosis. *J Nat Cancer Inst* 1971;47:747-756.
111. Watkins LR, Hutchinson MR, Ledeboer H, et al. Glia as the "bad guys": implications for improving clinical pain control and the utility of opioids. *Brain Behav Immun* 2007;21:131-146.
112. Watkins LR, Maier SF. Beyond neurons: evidence that immune and glial cells contribute to pathologic pain states. *Physiol Rev* 2002;82:981-1011.
113. Wood PB, Glabus MF, Simpson R, et al. Changes in gray matter density in fibromyalgia: correlation with dopamine metabolism. *J Pain* 2009;10:609-618.
114. Zang Y, Chee A, Shi P, et al. Intervertebral disc cells produce interleukins found in patients with back pain. *Am J Phys Med* 2016;95:407-415.
115. Zhang N, Zou Y, Jiang L, et al. Epstein Barr virus and neurologic diseases. *Front Mol Biosci* 2022;10:1-34.
116. Zweiman B, Levinson AI. Immunologic aspects of neurological and neuromuscular diseases. *JAMA* 1992;268:2918-2922.

Index

OTHER BOOKS BY FOREST TENNANT

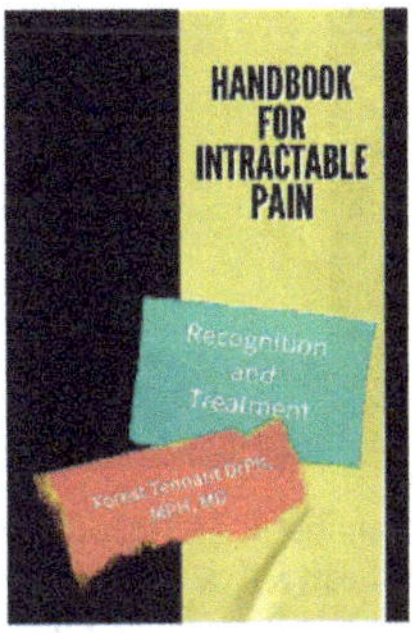

Handbook For Intractable Pain

ISBN:9781955934329
LOC:2023921074

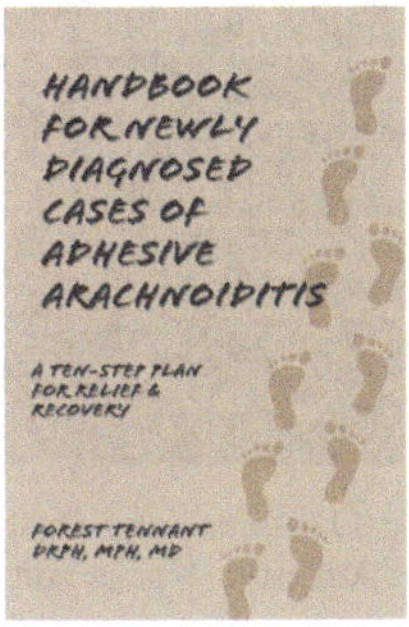

Handbook For Newly Diagnosed Cases of Adhesive Arachnoiditis

ISBN:9781955934244
LOC:2023908116

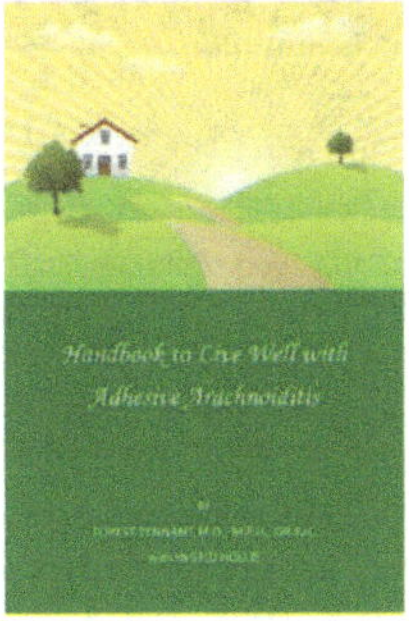

Handbook to Live Well with Adhesive Arachnoiditis

ISBN 978195934060
LOC: 2021912718

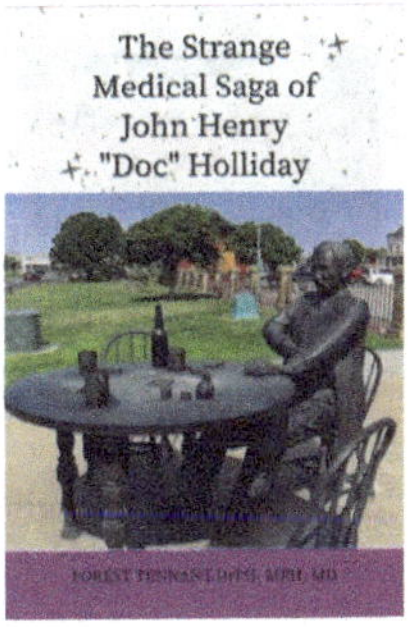

The Strange Medical Saga of John Henry "Doc Holiday"

ISBN:9781955934275
LOC 2023913628

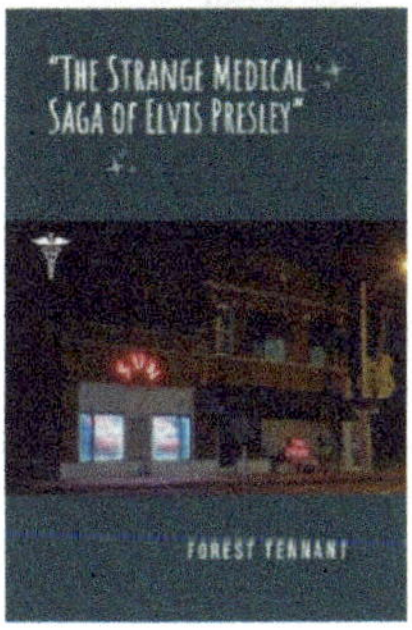

The Strange Medical Saga of Elvis Presley

ISBN: 9781955934008
LOC: 2021911718

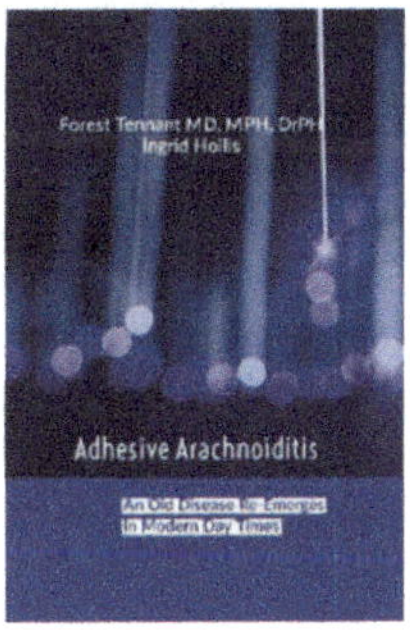

An Old Disease Re-Emerges in Modern Times

ISBN:9781955934039
LOC:2021912467

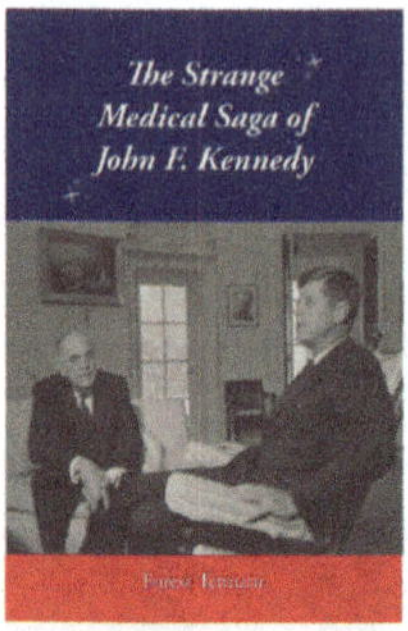

The Strange Medical Saga of John F. Kennedy

ISBN:9781955934213
LOC:2023903440

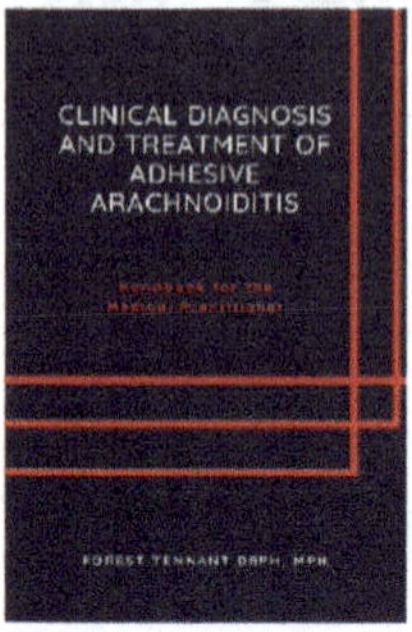

Clinical Diagnosis and Treatment of Adhesive Arachnoiditis

ISBN: 9781955934183
LOC: 2022907190

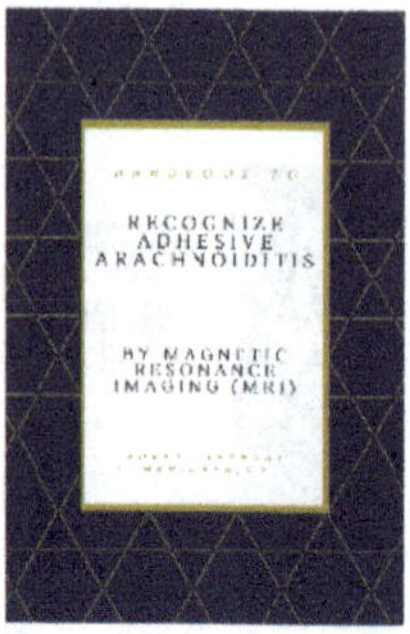

Handbook To Recognize Adhesive Arachnoiditis by Magnetic Resonance Imaging (MRI)

ISBN: 9781955934152
LOC: 2021925161

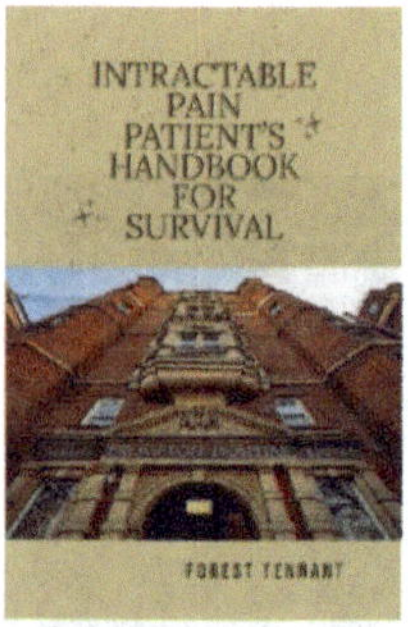

Intractable Pain Patients Handbook for Survival

ISBN: 9781955934121
LOC: 2021916464

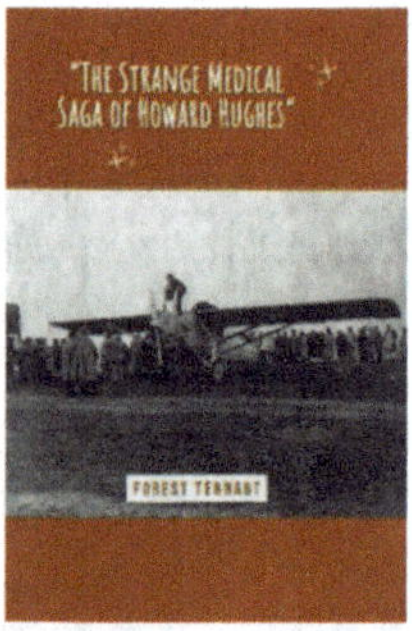

The Strange Medical Saga of Howard Hughes

ISBN: 9781955934091
LOC: 2021912855

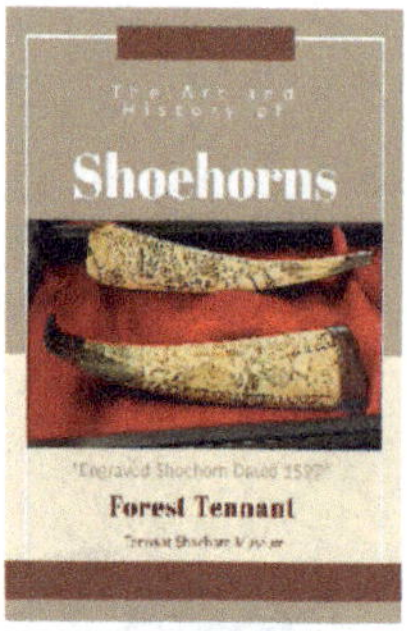

The Art and History of Shoehorns

ISBN:9781955934350
LOC:2024903219

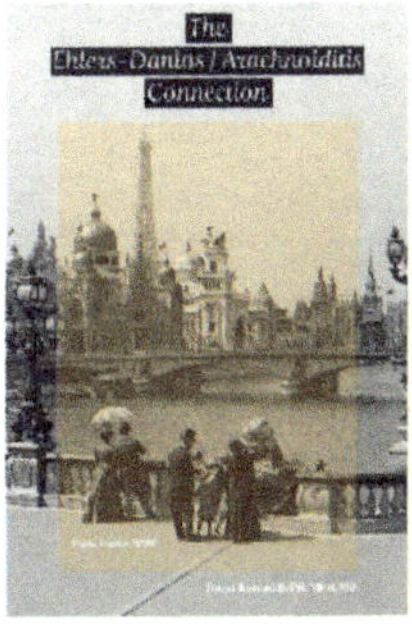

The Ehlers-Danlos /
Arachnoiditis Connenction

ISBN :9781955934381
LOC :2024911409

Made in United States
North Haven, CT
11 November 2026

22113773R00075